Alzheimer's, Memory Loss, and MCI

The Latest Science for Prevention & Treatment

David Leonardi, MD
Nathan Daley, MD, MPH

ISBN: 1470030470
ISBN-13: 9781470030476
Library of Congress Control Number: 2012902904
CreateSpace, North Charleston, SC

Table of Contents

FOREWORD   Mimi Guarneri, MD, FACC v

INTRODUCTION vii

PART ONE   THE PROBLEM AND THE SOLUTION 1

Chapter 1   Six Steps to Prevent and Treat Alzheimer's
            Disease 1
            How and Why Our Program Works

Chapter 2   Winning With the Hand You Were Dealt 13
            Using Knowledge as Motivation

PART TWO   BUILDING A BETTER BRAIN 19

Step 1   "Rustproofing" 19
         Limit Oxidative Stress

Step 2   Prevent "Sticky" Proteins 37
         Limit Glycation

Step 3   Make Your Genes Work in Your Favor 49
         The Magic of the Multisupplement

Step 4   Combat the Root Causes of Alzheimer's Disease. 57
          Protect and Defend Your Brain

Step 5   The Importance of Hormones for Your Brain. 89
          Safely Maintaining Healthy Hormone Levels

Step 6   Improve Your Brain Power. .103
          Brain Aerobics, Meditation & Sleep

Closing Note from the Authors   Back in the Driver's Seat. 119
          The Results Depend on Your Efforts

Appendix   Why Bioidentical Hormone Replacement
            Therapy for Menopause Is Safe 129

References. 135

Index 171

Foreword

Western medicine excels in the treatment of acute conditions. Whether it is the management of a heart attack or the need for trauma surgery, Western medicine provides state-of-the-art, frequently lifesaving treatment. Problems result when the acute care model is used to prevent and treat chronic disease. As physicians we are taught to make a diagnosis and recommend a treatment. Symptoms lead to a diagnosis that can in turn be billed, classified, and acted upon. What results is the "ill to the pill" model of healthcare in which each diagnosis exists in a silo with a treatment attached. The end result is what we currently have, a $310 billion pharmaceutical industry. What is lacking in this approach is a simple question, "What is the underlying cause of the problem in the first place?" Depression is a perfect example to illustrate this thinking. Once a diagnosis of depression is made, antidepressants are frequently prescribed. But the causes of depression are multiple. Depression may be situational, or related to seasonal affective disorder or low vitamin D. Antidepressants are not the treatment for all three of these causes.

Our Western medical model needs to shift from a silo approach in which we have diseases and specialists to a functional medicine systems approach in which we address the final common pathways and underlying causes of disease. For example, heart disease has many causes, including oxidative stress and inflammation. These same pathways lead to Alzheimer's disease and arthritis. By thinking in systems, we can quickly appreciate that what benefits one condition will benefit the others as well.

If a tree is sick we have a choice: we can cut off the fruit and branches or we can strengthen the soil. Our human soil can best be thought of from an epigenetic perspective. Each of us has twenty-three chapters in our book of life—the chromosomes we inherit from our parents. But we know that our genes are not our destiny. Genetically identical twins do not manifest the same diseases later in life. What washes over our genes determines whether we stay healthy or manifest disease. How we live our lives, what we eat, physical activity, environmental toxins, and our connection to people and the planet are just a few of the factors that turn our genes on and off. Research by Dr. Dean Ornish in men with prostate cancer shows that four hundred cancer promoter genes can be turned off through lifestyle change. Daily exercise trumps the obesity gene, for example.

Alzheimer's disease, like cardiac disease, is complex. Unfortunately, we do not have a single "magic bullet" for treating dementia and loss of cognitive function. Dr. Daley and Dr. Leonardi offer a systems approach to strengthening our soil through lifestyle change choices that are practical yet powerful. As with cardiovascular disease, macro and micro nutrition, physical activity, responses to stress and tension, and proper supplementation are some of the key ingredients to optimal health. The steps we implement to reduce oxidative stress and decrease inflammation benefit not only the brain but the heart, gastrointestinal system, and skeletal muscle system as well. These same steps will improve insulin resistance, diabetes, high blood pressure, and elevated cholesterol. The path to health is truly not that complex. Dr. Daley and Dr. Leonardi offer a compelling, well-thought-out, evidence-based roadmap.

Mimi Guarneri MD FACC

Founder and Medical Director
Scripps Center for Integrative Medicine

Introduction

The current disease care system is broken, inefficient, and expensive. Furthermore, the disease-oriented paradigm that underlies this system is ineffective in preventing or treating most degenerative diseases, including Alzheimer's disease. It is inevitable that the current system will change, but it is uncertain whether this change will result from a catastrophic collapse or an intelligent transition, led by innovative and thoughtful healers, toward a better medicine. We are optimistic that the latter scenario is possible, and this hope is supported by a growing population of physicians and other health-care providers who are offering patients a new approach to disease and a real chance at true health. This book was written in the spirit of facilitating this transition toward a better, more complete medicine. In the pages that follow, we provide the basic details of a new and comprehensive approach, synthesized from the work of thousands of researchers, to prevent and treat Alzheimer's disease. We offer this information to the general public, people with normal age-related memory impairment, those with mild cognitive impairment (MCI), Alzheimer's patients, and innovative health-care providers with the hope of improving lives and expanding medicine.

David Leonardi, MD
Nathan Daley, MD, MPH

PART ONE: THE PROBLEM AND THE SOLUTION

✤

Chapter 1

Six Steps to Prevent and Treat Alzheimer's Disease

How and Why Our Program Works

"Whatever you can do, or dream you can, begin it.
Boldness has genius, power and magic in it."

Johann Wolfgang von Goethe (1749–1832)

If we didn't know what to do about Alzheimer's disease (AD), our best choice might be to accept it and resign ourselves to the gradual deterioration with an attitude of "Don't worry, be happy." But we *do* know what to do. The work of many brilliant scientists around the world shows us that we can extend our quality of life and live longer if we're willing to invest in our own health.

At the Leonardi Institute, we have created a six-step plan that incorporates the most effective and promising results of decades of research. And we've combined these powerful approaches in a way that they enhance one another to produce the best possible outcomes.

As Aristotle wisely said, "The whole is greater than the sum of its parts." And for that reason, it's critical for you to follow all six steps rather than picking and choosing a few and disregarding the others.

What's in It for You?

▶ If you have a normal brain, you can maintain your optimal brain function and even improve your brain going forward.

▶ If you have mild cognitive impairment (MCI or pre-Alzheimer's), or you or a loved one has AD, you can slow, arrest, or possibly (we believe probably) improve your brain function.

What Is Your Brain State?

While some have already received a definitive diagnosis from a qualified physician, there are millions of people in mid-life who are experiencing some degree of cognitive difficulty and are wondering if they should be concerned. It's now fairly easy to find out. In our fifties—or sooner—we all experience those "senior moments" when we forget a familiar name, find ourselves word-searching in mid-sentence, walk into a room only to question why we did, or misplace items. For most of us this is due to normal age-related memory impairment, or simply distraction. For too many, however, these lapses can represent the tip of the iceberg: a condition called mild cognitive impairment or MCI. MCI is very different from normal age-related memory loss because it results from the same pathologic process as Alzheimer's disease – the accumulation of beta amyloid plaque in the brain (much more on this below). In fact, MCI is considered pre-Alzheimer's. Ten percent of people with MCI will progress on to Alzheimer's each year. Doing the math, it would follow that 100 percent of those with MCI today will have AD in ten years. But it's not that simple. A small percentage of those with MCI will not develop Alzheimer's and it's still not clear how to predict with great accuracy which MCI patients will progress to AD.

All of this can be sorted out with professional cognitive testing and an Amyvid PET scan. Together these tests can place you in the normal, MCI, or Alzheimer's dementia category. At the Leonardi Institute, we rely heavily on both of these tests, not only to diagnose accurately but also to provide a quantitative baseline by which to measure progress with our program. Just FDA approved at the time of this writing, the Amyvid PET scan is the first imaging study that can accurately measure the amount of beta amyloid plaque in the brain. Beta amyloid plaque accumulates even before cognition declines, so the Amyvid scan alerts us to the presence of impending AD early, when we have the best chance to arrest the disease process. Whichever category you fall into: normal, MCI, or Alzheimer's dementia, our six-step program is designed to improve your brain function going forward.

How It Works

Our Six-Step Program is explained in detail in this book. For each step, we explain what you need to do and why it works. We keep the scientific explanations as basic as possible to make them easier to read and comprehend. While some readers may be tempted to skip these explanations, we encourage you to read them. Understanding how and why our recommendations work will give you faith in the program and motivate you to invest the time and energy to incorporate each step into your daily life. From our combined forty years of practicing medicine, we've learned that people are far better at making healthy changes when they understand why they should.

We want our patients to make wise decisions based on reliable information, and we want the same for you. When you understand the science, you can see why doing what we suggest is worth the effort. This will strengthen your commitment, which in turn will produce better results. Your success depends on your level of effort, and for most people that's proportional to the degree of belief in what they're doing. We're not asking for blind faith. We're suggesting that you read the evidence from published clinical trials included in this book.

This approach empowers *you* to take control and become your own healer. The word *doctor*, after all, comes from the Latin *docere*, which means "to teach." Health and healing come from within and begin with information and understanding.

Why It Works

If you ask any physician, he or she will tell you that Alzheimer's disease has no cure and is invariably fatal.

We feel very differently about Alzheimer's. Doctors believe there is no cure because we don't yet have a magic bullet in the form of a single drug to stop or reverse the brain deterioration. The reason is that drug treatment can target only a single chemical reaction in the body. As an example, antibiotics block a single chemical reaction required by bacteria to live, and the effect is dramatic. But Alzheimer's is a very different animal; its causes are many. So, unlike treating strep throat, targeting one single chemical reaction won't work. For the most part, the FDA-approved medications for Alzheimer's disease merely increase the production of the neurotransmitter acetylcholine in the brain for a temporary improvement in cognition while the underlying disease progresses. The only exception to this statement is the drug memantine (Namenda), which works by a different mechanism but whose effect is nonetheless only temporary.

The key to controlling this disease is examining all the biochemistry we know of and taking a multifaceted approach to alter that biochemistry. Brilliant scientists have handed us reams of information in thousands of published studies; while there is much more to learn, the biochemistry of Alzheimer's is now significantly understood. But no one has attempted to simultaneously influence all the pathways by which Alzheimer's develops, let alone assembled the elements to block each pathway and clean up the mess that's in the brain—until now.

That's exactly what we've done, and in this book we give you a comprehensive treatment program that we believe is extremely effective. Our treatment program is not a single pill; to have a real effect on Alzheimer's, we have to use multiple elements. Our program consists of about thirty elements, which include lifestyle modification, specific nutritional supplements, bioidentical hormones, and specific prescription medications. (In Steps 1 through 6 we'll examine the biochemical events that lead to the plaques, tangles, and death of brain cells. We'll introduce you to each of the elements we discovered that interfere with and mitigate those biochemical events so you can take advantage of as many as possible.) In other words, controlling your disease will require some effort on your part.

If you're now taking or plan to take one of the FDA-approved medications for Alzheimer's, you should know that this program will not interfere with that medication and you may continue it while following this program.

Your Brain's "Anti-Alzheimer's" Avenues

Imagine the map of a city where nine avenues lead directly to the city center like nine spokes on a wheel. Now picture your brain as the city center. In Alzheimer's disease, the brain is attacked along seven of these avenues at once. The other two avenues are supply routes for nurturing and improving your brain. Arresting or reversing AD requires keeping your two supply avenues open while defending the brain from enemies attacking via the other seven avenues. To be successful, we must tend to all nine avenues simultaneously.

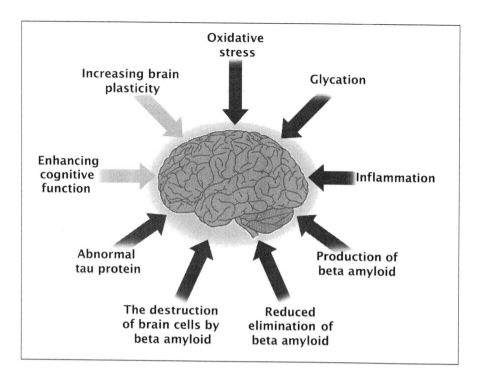

Oxidative stress

Increasing brain plasticity

Glycation

Enhancing cognitive function

Inflammation

Abnormal tau protein

Production of beta amyloid

The destruction of brain cells by beta amyloid

Reduced elimination of beta amyloid

While drug companies and universities search for the magic bullet, thousands of published studies that shed light on the root causes of AD are sitting in the National Library of Medicine. Many other studies provide evidence that specific elements of therapy are effective against these root causes. And some of these elements have actually been shown to benefit Alzheimer's patients in placebo-controlled clinical trials. Not a single one by itself has been able to effect a cure. That's because each one defends against one, two, or several avenues of attack on the brain, but none covers all nine. However, combining all these elements *does* cover all seven avenues of attack and our two supply avenues. Amazingly enough though, no one has ever assembled all these weapons into a workable program. Our approach is to do just that.

As you read about the six steps in our plan, you'll be introduced to multiple therapeutic weapons against AD. Each of these weapons has a specific function that targets one or more of the avenues by which your brain is being attacked.

Some of these weapons provide a defense, and some deliver a counterattack. Each weapon has a critically important purpose. Each, in and of itself is extremely beneficial, but it's our *combination of these weapons* that will likely prevent, probably arrest, and quite possibly even reverse AD.

The Seven Avenues to Alzheimer's Disease

Avenue 1: Oxidative Stress

Oxidative stress kills brain cells, and levels of oxidative stress are increased in the brains of people with AD; this stress may lead to brain plaque. It may also be related to the accumulation of abnormal tau protein, which leads to tangling of the tubules in brain cells and, ultimately, cell death. Yet even if oxidative stress doesn't directly promote these two processes, it certainly works along with them to kill brain cells.

There is also a likely connection between oxidative stress and the dysfunction of important structures in brain cells called mitochondria. Mitochondria are the power plants of all cells, and dysfunction at the power plants translates to energy deficiency and dysfunction of the entire brain cell.

Avenue 2: Glycation

Glycation is the bonding of sugar to protein. It is a normal but harmful process that is discussed in detail in Step 2. When sugar in our body bonds permanently to a protein, the protein is referred to as glycated.

Combating glycation is an important step in arresting or reversing AD. Glycated proteins are found in higher levels in the Alzheimer's brain and are also found in the plaques and tangles. Glycation occurs at the highest known level in diabetes, and diabetics have an increased risk of AD. Excessive glycation also promotes more oxidative stress (Avenue 1).

Avenue 3: Inflammation

As oxidative stress and glycation create destructive molecules in our bodies and brains, our immune system attempts to get rid of the troublemakers. Our white blood cells wage a chemical war on these molecules much as they would against a virus or bacteria. The name for this war is *inflammation*. And, as in all war, there is collateral damage. The collateral damage to our normal cells and tissue from this chemical attack by our immune system leads to further loss of brain cells.

Avenue 4: Production of Beta-Amyloid Protein in the Brain

The brains of Alzheimer's patients don't get rid of excess beta-amyloid protein fast enough, so it accumulates, and this accumulation eventually kills brain cells. It's like a sink with the faucet running and the drain blocked; to prevent overflow, we open the drain and slow the water flowing out of the faucet. Our attack on Avenue 4 is the reduction of beta-amyloid production, akin to slowing flow from the faucet.

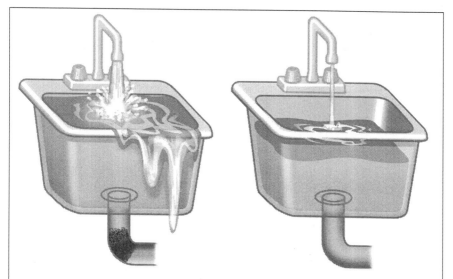

Brain overload of beta amyloid protein is due to reduced elimination, somewhat like a plugged sink might overload the bowl. To combat or prevent this most effectively, we both reduce production of beta amyloid (analogous to reducing flow from the faucet) and enhance elimination of beta amyloid (analogous to opening the drain). If elimination can keep up with production we reach a healthy state.

Avenue 5: Reduced Elimination of Beta-Amyloid Protein in the Brain

Elimination of beta–amyloid protein (opening the drain) can be accelerated by two main mechanisms. Immune cells called macrophages can gobble it up, engulfing and digesting it like Pac-Man. Or enzymes can break it down. There are three known enzymes that do this: insulin-degrading enzyme (IDE), transthyretin, and neprilysin.

Some of the thirty elements of our program stimulate macrophages to engulf and digest beta amyloid, and some stimulate one or more of the three enzymes that break it down.

Avenue 6: Destruction of Brain Cells by Beta-Amyloid Toxicity

This destruction is well demonstrated in dozens of studies. However, there also exists a time period before destruction in which the brain cell does not function normally, contributing to cognitive impairment even though the brain cell is still alive. This dysfunctional state is probably reversible, and therefore brain-cell function and cognitive function can be improved. Our program protects brain cells from the dysfunction and death caused by beta-amyloid toxicity.

Avenue 7: Abnormal Tau Protein

Tau protein is an important component of the structures in our brain cells called tubules, which are like steel beams that provide structural support. In Alzheimer's disease abnormal chemistry causes the tau protein strands to break, causing the tubules to bend and tangle, much like melted steel. When this happens, brain cells lose their structural supports and die. Many of our program elements protect tau protein from being broken, in turn protecting the tubules and the brain cells from destruction.

Defending Attack and Fortifying Our Supply Avenues

To defend these seven avenues of attack, we'll be using all the elements that scientists have found to be effective in protecting the brain from each one. We believe that if we can reduce oxidative stress and glycation, inhibit the production of beta amyloid, speed up the removal of beta amyloid, protect brain cells from the beta amyloid already present, and protect the tau protein from destruction, we can at least arrest and possibly reverse the disease process.

In addition to defending the seven avenues of attack, we must also keep our two supply avenues open. This ensures that our brains get all the nutrition and other supplements they need to enhance cognitive function and improve the ability of brain circuitry to rewire itself, a process known as plasticity. While there is some overlap between the following two avenues (8 and 9), they are not identical processes.

Avenue 8: Enhancing Cognitive Function

Many of the elements in our program have been shown in clinical trials to enhance brain cell performance, not just by squeezing more neurotransmitters from the brain cell but by nurturing and protecting it. The benefits in clinical trials have largely been short-term, but our expectation is that by using all thirty elements together, we can accomplish long-term improvement in cognition.

Avenue 9: Improving Plasticity

Plasticity is the development of new brain cells and the development of new connections between brain cells. Many of our program elements have been shown in scientific studies to accomplish both of these tasks. Improving plasticity leads to a smarter and more functional brain.

The Key to Your Success

We want to be very clear about this: We don't want to mislead anyone into believing that using one, two, or ten of the thirty elements in our program will make a significant difference in the outcome of any case of Alzheimer's disease. We believe that if our program is to be truly successful in arresting or reversing the disease, all—or at least a vast majority—of the thirty elements must be applied simultaneously. On the other hand, it wouldn't surprise us if employing some of the elements provided modest benefits in slowing the disease's progression. So if that's all you're able to manage, we encourage you to do so. Every bit of effort you can invest is worth it, because the only other option is to let your brain deteriorate while you receive palliative care.

The required effort is significant but far from overwhelming. We'll teach you everything you need to know in this short book. We encourage you to embrace the information in this book and become an expert on it. Then apply all the elements we prescribe. We believe you'll be greatly rewarded for your effort.

PLEASE NOTE: If you think you're cognitively impaired, we encourage you to enlist the help of a family member or friend who can help you obtain all the necessary materials, perform all the necessary functions, partner with a good doctor, and monitor your progress.

Chapter 2

Winning With the Hand
You Were Dealt

Using Knowledge as Motivation

When people are diagnosed with Alzheimer's disease, they often feel devastated and afraid. They feel as if their future and all their hopes and dreams have just been snatched away. They worry that they will be a burden to their loved ones but dread the idea of being in a long-term care facility. All these reactions and many more cast a dark shadow and make the future look bleak.

There is no doubt that AD is a horrible disease, but you have the power to slow the progression of the disease and possibly even reverse it. And now you have the knowledge, too. Your challenge is to win with the hand you were dealt. Of course, it's not a hand you would have chosen, but by taking the steps we've laid out in this book, you can make a profound difference in your own health and longevity. The last thing we want you to do is fold.

If a loved one has been diagnosed with AD, encourage him or her to read this book and see how much power they truly have to slow or reverse this disease.

How Alzheimer's Disease Progresses Without Adequate Treatment

Alzheimer's disease is a devastating dementia resulting in loss of multiple brain functions having to do with cognition (thought). Initially, short-term memory is most affected, resulting in the inability to have a normal conversation. Patients may ask questions repeatedly about simple things they were just told.

Loss of executive function typically comes next. Executive function is the ability to organize tasks and follow the organization of a described task or process. Examples would be balancing a checkbook and organizing errands in a logical manner, with a mental checklist that might look like this: Take Angie to school; stop at the market to pick up tomatoes, bread, and bananas; and drop off the bananas at Margaret's house on the way home. Appointments are forgotten, important household tasks are often omitted, and finances are mismanaged.

As the disease progresses, it becomes obvious to family members. Conversation is impaired when searching for a word takes so long that the initial concept of the sentence is forgotten. Activities of daily living such as dressing, bathing, housekeeping, and preparing meals become difficult or impossible.

Alzheimer's progresses at different rates in different people, and often the progression happens in fits and starts. One may be fairly stable for a number of months and then experience a rapid deterioration. Eventually, behavior is affected and Alzheimer's patients can become irritable, obstinate, and even combative. Some patients simply remain happily disabled, but more often there is some level of depression.

Ultimately, the disease progresses to a state of complete dependence and death if another cause of death does not intervene.

Alzheimer's disease is the sixth leading cause of death, with more than five million people in the United States alone currently suffering from the disease. Further, the nearly eleven million family members directly caring for these people are at a significantly elevated health risk due to the stress and strain that such care demands. The aging baby-boomer population will cause these figures to skyrocket.

So personally and nationally, we all have a vested interest in learning how to prevent and reverse Alzheimer's disease. But to do that, we have to have some understanding of what causes it.

What's Going on in the Brain?

We don't want to dwell on the negative aspects of this disease, but we do want you to understand what's happening in the brain so you can understand how and why our Six-Step Plan works.

We're pleased to say that thanks to scientific research, the causes of AD are becoming clearer. We've learned that the loss of brain cells is due to the toxicity of two components that accumulate in the brain: beta-amyloid protein and neurofibrillary tangles.

Beta-Amyloid Protein

We used to think beta-amyloid protein was an abnormal protein formed in the brains of Alzheimer's patients. But now we know that it's a normal protein that accumulates in their brains because their brains are clearing it out too slowly. It's not the protein itself that causes problems—it's having an excess amount of the protein. When too much of it builds up, it becomes toxic to the brain.

Brain cells function by conducting electrical impulses much like an electric wire. These electric impulses cause the cell to release neurotransmitters, or signaling chemicals, that drift over to the next cell to start an impulse there. This is how brain cells work together in a network. Through that network, our thoughts are created, memories are stored and retrieved, vision and hearing are processed, and our movement is controlled. In a normally functioning brain, beta-amyloid protein suppresses certain brain-cell activity to prevent the cells from firing too many impulses too quickly, which could create chaos.

An excess of beta-amyloid protein "oversuppresses" brain-cell activity, damaging cells and the connections among cells. As this protein accumulates, it also causes oxidation—the brain-cell "rusting" we will discuss in Step 1. Eventually, the brain cell dies. And the more brain cells that die, the more brain function declines. In Alzheimer's disease, brain-cell death is most prominent in the area of the brain that we use for memory. This area, called the hippo-campus, is on the sides of the brain, close to the tops of the ears, in the temporal lobe.

When Alzheimer's brains are examined at autopsy, large amounts of beta-amyloid protein are found accumulated in pods or deposits called plaque (beta-amyloid plaque). This plaque is found in areas of brain atrophy (shrinkage). The atrophy is caused, very simply, by the loss of the brain cells that have been destroyed by the beta-amyloid protein and other destructive processes.

Neurofibrillary Tangles

Neurofibrillary tangles are formed when normal structures in the brain cell called tubules are deformed. Tubules are supported by a protein component called tau. In Alzheimer's patients, the tau protein is chemically altered so that it is unable to physically support the structural rigidity of the tubules. As a result, the tubules become curled and tangled, thus the term *neurofibrillary tangles*.

It was recently discovered that some people accumulate beta-amyloid plaque without losing brain function. This is because they don't have the abnormal tau protein and neurofibrillary tangles. So it appears that the accumulation of beta-amyloid plaque and neurofibrillary tangles work together to kill brain cells in Alzheimer's cases. And that's why in our Six-Step Program, we give both of these causes equal attention.

Why There's No "One" Cure

For decades, research has been focused on the biochemical processes that create beta-amyloid plaque and neurofibrillary tangles in hopes of finding a single drug that can alter a single chemical reaction to arrest the disease. Unfortunately, success at this game is a long shot, which is why billions of research dollars spent over several decades have not resulted in a pharmaceutical solution. Why, then, would drug companies take this approach? Remember, drug companies are like every other company: they are businesses whose plan is to be financially successful. This is dependent on their creating the next blockbuster drug—a magic bullet, if you will, that can be patented and will effect a cure for a devastating disease, bringing in billions of dollars. And major universities aren't much different. Their research departments are always hungry for funding. So their focus is similar to that of drug companies, and alliances are often formed to share research and then revenue when the FDA approves a drug they discovered together.

Alzheimer's disease has so far proved to be too complex for a single pharmaceutical cure. The accumulation of beta-amyloid plaque and neurofibrillary tangles is more complex than a single chemical reaction creating each. That's why it's unlikely that a single drug that blocks a single chemical reaction will ever cure AD. Even if one is discovered tomorrow, it will take years to go through the test tube and animal and human studies to demonstrate safety and efficacy.

So rather than cross our fingers and hope, we teach our patients how to do everything in their power to combat this disease. And remember, when we work at the lifestyle level, we can have a dramatic impact on all the root causes of AD that we currently know about. The purpose of this book is to teach you what we teach our patients.

✤

PART TWO

BUILDING A BETTER BRAIN

STEP 1 "Rustproofing"
Limit Oxidative Stress

When I was a young boy, I saw my first example of oxidative stress. It was a rusted cast-iron skillet. I remember wondering what made it rust, since nothing else in my grandmother's attic was rusted. Later I learned that oxygen can make iron rust. If the skillet had been protected with oil, it would have been sealed off from the oxygen and resistant to rust. The rusting process is called oxidative stress. It happens when one element causes destructive change to another. In this case, the oxygen destructively changed the iron surface of the skillet.

When oxidative stress occurs in our bodies, it damages our cells and can eventually damage our organs, including our brains. Everyone should limit oxidative stress, but for people who are at higher risk for Alzheimer's disease or already have the disease, this is a critically important step. In this chapter you will learn what promotes oxidative stress and how you can combat it. Our primary goal for Step 1 is to reduce the level of oxidative stress in your brain.

The Science of Oxidative Stress and Free Radicals

Oxidative stress is a normal but destructive process that occurs constantly in all of us. It is associated with aging and deterioration of the human organism. There is abundant evidence that the Alzheimer's brain undergoes higher levels of oxidative stress than a normal brain and that oxidative stress is responsible for much of the damage and brain-cell death that occurs with Alzheimer's disease.[1–5] That said, what is oxidative stress and what can we do to control it?

Oxidative stress involves the production of *oxygen free radicals.* Very simply, a free radical is an atom with an unpaired electron. Our bodies are composed of billions of cells. Cells are biochemical structures composed of many molecules. Molecules, in turn, are made of atoms. Free radicals are formed at the level of atoms. An atom has a nucleus that contains protons, and this nucleus is orbited by electrons.

Electrons are like people. They like to travel in pairs. An electron that is orbiting the nucleus all by itself is a free radical. It will do anything it can to get a mate. So what it does is jump ship to the next atom, knock an electron out of its orbit and take its mate. Then the electron that got knocked out is the free radical, and it immediately goes to the next atom, knocks an electron out of its orbit and takes its mate, and so on.

What we end up with is a rapid-fire transfer of electrons, and every time an electron transfer occurs, there is a potential structural change in the molecule. Structural change in a molecule is equivalent to molecular damage. This is one of the main mechanisms by which we lose brain cells as we age, and it occurs in spades in people with Alzheimer's disease.

Cells can withstand only so many insults by free radicals interfering with their normal metabolism. When a certain number of free radicals assault a neuron (brain cell), it will literally self-destruct and die. In people with Alzheimer's disease, the beta-amyloid protein increases free radical formation, and that is one of the ways that beta amyloid is toxic to brain cells.[6–11] The normal causes of oxidative stress combine with beta amyloid to hasten the loss of brain cells, resulting in the excessive brain atrophy seen in AD.

Avoiding Pro-Oxidant Metals

Certain metal elements called "pro-oxidants" are toxic to the brain because they rapidly promote oxidative stress. Because of their chemical structure, these metals promote free-radical formation very rapidly and vigorously. These include aluminum,[12–19] mercury,[12, 20–25] copper,[26–31] and iron, when in excess.[32–37]

By limiting our brains' exposure to these four metals, we can slow the attrition of our brain cells. This is critically important in Alzheimer's disease; all four of these metals have been found in higher levels in AD brains than normal brains. To reduce our brain's exposure to these destructive metals, we must look at each separately.

Aluminum

Aluminum is one of the easiest of the four metals to avoid. One of the major sources of aluminum exposure is processed foods and mixes, such as pancake or waffle mix and baking powder. In fact, the average amount of aluminum in one serving of pancake mix can easily exceed the dose that, when given to rats, contributed to the development of AD.[32, 33]

While premade mixes save time in the short run, they can cost you years of trouble in the long run. There are plenty of recipes for making your own mixes, and they are all relatively fast and easy.

Aluminum is found in all antiperspirants (not deodorants). AD patients and those who wish to prevent AD should avoid antiperspirants.

Do not use aluminum cookware or cook with aluminum foil. Even covering a baking dish with aluminum foil is probably harmful. Water boils in the dish, evaporates, and condenses on the foil, only to drip back onto the food with traces of aluminum.

Water treated with alum is common in many municipal water supplies; the alum is used to precipitate solid waste from the water in the treatment process. Find out if aluminum is being used in your municipality. Most large cities supply this information, but you may have to dig a bit to find it. Type the following into the search box on Google.com or your preferred search engine: *Name of your city*, followed by *municipal water treatment.* (For example: *Denver municipal water treatment.*) If you can't find the information using this suggested search, call your city's facility to ask, or treat your drinking water with reverse osmosis as a precaution.

If alum is used in your city's water treatment, we strongly recommend drinking water processed by reverse osmosis or distillation. Installing a reverse-osmosis filter at the tap is generally the best option, but it can be costly and tends to waste water. Though not ideal, bottled water may be necessary. If you drink bottled water, pick a brand that is treated with either of these two processes. You may need to call the toll-free number on the bottle to determine the exact purification process. In a perfect world, this water would be provided in glass bottles to avoid additional contaminants from plastic, but this is not common practice. The following are two brands (there are probably others) that satisfy the reverse-osmosis or distillation criteria but are not sold in glass bottles: Nestle Pure Life (healthy minerals added after treatment with reverse osmosis) and Smart Water (healthy minerals added after distillation). These brands also provide the benefit of replacing important minerals that are removed by the purification process.

Immunizations are another source of aluminum. Metals are used to enhance the immune response to the microbial proteins present in vaccines. Aluminum is used due to its effectiveness and perceived safety (as compared with mercury, for example).

Immunizations are important for controlling infectious diseases, so complete avoidance is not recommended. The best approach to limiting aluminum exposure from vaccinations is to maintain very accurate records and avoid repeated and unnecessary vaccinations. Additionally, not all vaccines available to older adults are necessary for each individual, so an informed discussion with your physician to determine what may be appropriate for you can also help eliminate unnecessary exposure.

Mercury

Mercury is bad for our brain and our nervous system. Ask your health-care provider to test the mercury level in your blood. While there is controversy over how representative this test is of your brain mercury level, it nonetheless serves as a barometer to let you know about how much mercury you are carrying. Two of the biggest sources of mercury are fishes that are high in mercury and dental fillings that contain mercury.

If you've been eating fish that has high or moderate levels of mercury, it's time to switch to the lower-mercury choices. The ocean's largest predator fishes are highest in mercury, because they have accumulated mercury from many years of eating smaller fish that have ingested mercury.

The following is a partial list from the Natural Resources Defense Council website.

High Mercury—Do Not Eat These Fish!

▶ Bluefish grouper

▶ Mackerel (Spanish, gulf)

▶ Mackerel (king)

▶ Marlin

▶ Orange roughy

▶ Sea bass (Chilean)

▶ Shark

▶ Swordfish

▶ Tilefish

▶ Tuna (bigeye, ahi, yellowfin, canned albacore)

Moderate Mercury—Limit Intake to Three per Month

► Bass (striped, black)

► Carp cod (Alaskan)

▷ Croaker (white Pacific)

▷ Halibut (Atlantic)

▷ Halibut (Pacific)

▷ Lobster

▷ Mahi mahi

▷ Monkfish

▷ Perch (freshwater)

▷ Skate

► Snapper

► Tuna (canned chunk light)

Lowest Mercury—Eat as Often as You Like

▷ Anchovies

► Butterfish

► Catfish

► Clams

► Crab (domestic)

► Crawfish/Crayfish

► Flounder

► Haddock (Atlantic)

▶ Herring

▶ Mackerel (N. Atlantic, chub)

▶ Mullet

▶ Oyster

▶ Perch (ocean)

▶ Salmon (wild)*

▶ Sardines

▶ Scallops

▶ Shad (American)

▶ Shrimp

▶ Sole (Pacific

▶ Squid (calamari)

▶ Tilapia

▶ Trout (freshwater)

▶ Whitefish

▶ Whiting

*Farmed salmon and other farmed fish may contain PCBs, chemicals with serious long-term health effects. Most farmed fish should be avoided, not because of mercury content but because of PCBs and other toxins.

This list can change over time, so check the list at the Natural Resources Defense Council website (http://www.nrdc.org/health/effects/mercury/guide.asp) every year for updates. The NRDC provides a comprehensive list of seafood categorized by mercury content. It also makes recommendations on how often to eat those in each category, from lowest to highest mercury content.

The most important thing to do for mercury avoidance is to ask your doctor to check your serum mercury level. If it is above 8, avoid fish and seafood for one month and then resume at a level of intake lower than your previous level. Have your serum mercury level rechecked at least twice a year.

Dental Fillings

The compounds used to fill cavities (dental amalgams) sometimes contain mercury. If you have AD or are at high risk, we strongly advise having these amalgams removed. But don't just go to any dentist for this procedure. Do your homework by making sure that the dentist you choose to do the work is qualified in a technique that uses suction and an air dam to prevent inhalation of the mercury vapor during the procedure. The mercury vapor is far more toxic than the fillings themselves! Have the amalgams replaced with a mercury-free substance, or protect the tooth with a gold crown.

Copper

Copper is another pro-oxidant. We typically get copper from food and drinking water, but nutritional supplements also contain copper, so we can easily get too much.

Copper from Food

Dietary copper is most abundant in organ meats (liver), shellfish, nuts, whole grains, concentrated tomato products, and mushrooms. With the exception of organ meats, these are generally healthful foods, and no restrictions are necessary when typical serving sizes are consumed. Organ meats, however, often contain excessive levels of copper (and iron) in addition to other potential contaminants and should generally be avoided.

Nutritional Supplements

Read the lists of ingredients on all nutritional supplements you are taking. If one or more of your supplements contain copper, make sure the total amount is no more than 0.4 mg (400 mcg) per day.

Water

If your home contains copper water pipes, you should begin treating your water using reverse osmosis or drink distilled water. Whether you have copper pipes or not, we recommend one of these two sources of drinking water for Alzheimer's patients.

However, keep in mind that distillation and reverse osmosis also remove beneficial minerals from water, such as calcium, magnesium, and potassium. When drinking distilled or reverse-osmosis-treated water, these minerals should be supplemented. The following table shows the recommended supplementation for people who drink water that is distilled or treated with reverse osmosis:

Calcium	800 mg per day
Potassium gluconate	1,000 mg per day (Equal to about 170 mg of *elemental* potassium, or about 4 milli-equivalents)
Magnesium amino acid chelate*	200 to 400 mg per day

*If you develop diarrhea, reduce the dosage of magnesium by 100 mg. If that doesn't stop the diarrhea, reduce it by another 50 mg.

CAUTION: If you have any type of compromised kidney function, check with your doctor before taking potassium or magnesium supplements.

Iron

A certain amount of iron is necessary to make healthy red blood cells and to prevent anemia. But when your body has too much iron, the excess iron promotes oxidative stress. It's important to find out how much iron your body is storing, and it's easy to do. Ask your health-care provider to order a blood test called serum ferritin. (Ferritin is the protein in our bodies that binds iron, so our ferritin levels reflect our total body iron levels.)

At most labs, the normal range is 20 to 380 ng/ml. But as we say at the Leonardi Institute, normal is often not optimal. We like to see ferritin levels from 20 to 100 ng/ml.

If your ferritin level is above 100 ng/ml, we recommend reducing it by donating blood. If you are not healthy enough to donate blood or have been rejected as a donor for other reasons, it's still important to reduce your iron level by having blood drawn and discarded. Your doctor can authorize a blood bank or a hospital to safely do this for you. How often and how much blood is drawn will be monitored to prevent iron-deficiency anemia. When your ferritin level drops below 50 ng/ml, you should stop donating blood or having it drawn and discarded until your ferritin level rises back above 100 ng/ml.

Avoiding foods that are high in iron can help keep your iron levels in the optimal range, but many of these foods are very healthy, so eliminating them usually isn't the best option. In the list below, we've underlined the specific items we believe you should continue to eat. Remember, you can balance your intake by donating blood.

Foods Highest in Iron

- ▶ Red meat

- ▶ Egg yolks

- ▶ <u>Dark, leafy greens</u>

- ▶ Dried fruit (raisins, prunes)

- ▶ Iron-enriched cereals and grains

► Mollusks (oysters, clams, scallops)

► Turkey or chicken giblets

► Beans, lentils, chickpeas, and soybeans

► Liver

► Artichokes

We recommend planning to donate blood regularly and not being too concerned about eating foods high in iron, particularly nonstarch vegetables and whole grains. The iron from these foods is not absorbed very efficiently, so it's hard to overdo it. The iron in red meat, on the other hand, is efficiently absorbed and should be minimized until your ferritin level is below 100 ng/dl.

Avoiding and "Binding" Toxic Metals

Aluminum, mercury, copper, iron, lead, and cadmium might also induce or promote Alzheimer's disease by means other than oxidation. Essentially, these metals may interact with beta-amyloid protein, a major culprit in Alzheimer's. This toxic interaction can actually destroy brain neurons.

The Science of Beta Amyloid

Information continues to flow regarding how these metal ions might interact with beta-amyloid protein in the brain, affecting not just its formation but the way the individual proteins aggregate together to form senile plaques and subsequently destroy neurons. One of the most likely mechanisms of such harmful interaction is oxidation – a destructive process involving transfer of electrons.[34–39] Aluminum, mercury, copper and iron have a strong tendency to promote oxidation in tissue, a property that designates them as "redox-positive". Although not considered redox-positive metals, lead and cadmium are implicated in the excessive *phosphorylation* (of tau protein and/or the accumulation of amyloid beta protein.[40–44] Phosphory-lation refers to the attachment of a phosphate chemical group to a molecule. Although this is a normal process in the body, when done to excess it causes the tau protein to weaken and break, leading to the neurofibrillary tangles (NFTs) that we've previously discussed.

Phytate (inositol hexaphosphate) binds metal ions, including redox-positive mercury, iron, and copper, and it binds iron and mercury preferentially over the minerals we prefer not be bound, such as magnesium, calcium, and potassium.[45–47] Phytate is also an efficient binder of lead and cadmium.[46] It has also been shown to reduce the production of beta-amyloid protein in the brain as well as protect neurons from amyloid toxicity.[36]

In addition to avoiding toxic metals, we must also bind or capture these ions in the blood and brain before they can do any damage. Binding all these metals can be extremely protective in the brain by limiting the high level of oxidation and other toxic reactions these metals generate. Fortunately, there is a nutrient called phytate that binds metal ions. Oat and rice bran are excellent sources of phytate. Lentils and dried beans contain phytate, too. The problem is that ingesting phytate can diminish our ability to absorb important nutrients like calcium, magnesium, and potassium. For that reason, we don't recommend an oral phytate *supplement,* but oat bran, rice bran, beans, and lentils are all healthy foods and should not be avoided.

To be sure our patients were getting enough phytate each day without impairing their ability to absorb other important nutrients from the intestine we developed a phytate cream for application to the skin. Our patients use one-quarter teaspoon of a 50 percent phytate cream daily, which supplies 625 mg of phytate. This is a good supplement to a typical daily oral intake of about 300 mg of phytate from food, and it ensures that the right level of phytate reaches the blood and the brain, where it will bind copper, iron, lead, cadmium, mercury, and aluminum ions. Phytate reduces oxidative stress and protects our brain cells from the other harm these metals can do.

Other Sources of Oxidative Stress

Air Pollution

Ideally, we want to avoid as much air pollution as possible, but unfortunately not many people have the freedom to pick up and move. So if you live in a big city or near a strong source of air pollution, like a coal-burning power plant, you'll need to be mindful of the outdoor air quality and time your outdoor activities accordingly.

By relying on up-to-the-minute information on your local air quality, you can plan to go outside when the pollution levels are at their lowest. Typically, the best air quality in cities is found just before morning rush hour, but seasonal exceptions may occur. You can get the latest air-quality information at www.airnow.gov. If you have AD, follow the recommendations for the "sensitive population." During times of peak air pollution, remain inside with filtered air as much as possible.

Use the highest-rated residential filters (i.e., MERV 10–12) in your home HVAC system. Free-standing HEPA-type filters are available and are also useful for further improving air quality in specific rooms. There are many reputable brands of HEPA filters available, and these are easily found with an Internet search, along with reviews of their performance.

When you're riding in a car, keep the ventilation system in the "recirculation" mode unless there is no other traffic on the road. This will circulate the air inside the car instead of pulling in the exhaust from the traffic around you. Even in light traffic, the outside air is loaded with carbon monoxide, diesel particulates, and other products of hydrocarbon combustion. When you inhale these compounds, they create inflammation throughout your body and spontaneously form oxygen free radicals.

Water Pollution

Earlier in this chapter we shared information about the alum in your drinking water. It's important to keep in mind that alum is not the only toxin found in water. Far from it. Everything from arsenic and lead to pharmaceutical drugs and hormone-disrupting chemicals may be pouring out of your faucets. For that reason, it's essential that you treat your drinking and cooking water properly and buy only water that is truly clean. Water quality and filtration are complex subjects. In general, tap water filtered by reverse osmosis (with mineral supplementation) is the most widely available healthy option for most people.

Pesticides

When we eat the pesticides that are on most vegetables and fruits, our liver and kidneys rapidly clear as much of them out of our bodies as possible. But this high-intensity cleaning job creates an army of oxygen free radicals, otherwise known as "the bad guys," because they increase oxidative stress. And although our bodies do an excellent job of "self-cleaning" when our liver processes the pesticides, some of the metabolic byproducts created in the process are toxic and remain active in our bodies.

Many pesticides contain ingredients that are highly toxic to our brains, called neurotoxins. Studies have shown that farmers, exterminators, chemical workers, and even gardeners who have low but chronic exposure to these chemicals have an increased incidence of AD. Many toxins in our world are very hard for us to avoid, but pesticides on produce is not one of them. We can *eliminate this danger to our brain by eating organic fruits and vegetables* and washing them well when we get them home. Most grocery stores spray for insects, and there is no law requiring them to cover the organic produce before they spray the area around it.

Electromagnetic Radiation or Fields (EMF)

Electromagnetic radiation is pervasive in most developed countries, giving rise to the term *electro-smog*. This type of radiation comes from electrical equipment, with wireless technologies creating a large portion of it. In general, the larger the motor or the greater the energy output, the greater the EMF. A number of studies have demonstrated an association between EMF exposure and AD incidence.[48] The mechanisms are less clear and probably multiple, including oxidative stress. The science quickly gets complicated, however, and it is uncertain which frequencies and amplitudes actually pose the greatest risk to our health.

EMF may also suppress our production of an important hormone called melatonin.[49] Melatonin can prevent several of the abnormal processes involved in AD. We cover this in more detail in Step 5, but for now start minimizing your exposure to EMF. This includes reducing your use of cell phones and other wireless technologies. The safest method of reducing EMF exposure when using your cell phone is to use the speaker phone or texting features. Also keep your proximity to operating electrical motors and appliances to the minimum amount that's reasonable. When it comes to any type of radiation, distance is your best friend.

What to Embrace

Organic Fruits and Vegetables

Not only should Alzheimer's patients eat *organic* produce, but they should eat lots of it because fruits and vegetables contain antioxidants. An antioxidant is a molecule that can collect a free radical (a rogue electron) and neutralize it before it can trigger another destructive cascade of electron transfers.

Antioxidants are specific nutrients such as beta carotene, vitamin E, vitamin C, alpha-lipoic acid, N-acetyl cysteine, coenzyme Q10, and selenium. Fruits and vegetables contain far, far more of these than animal foods. The more we neutralize free radicals, the greater the chance of preserving those brain cells we have left. Let them eat *organic* produce!

Antioxidant Supplements

While there are some conflicting studies, there is very strong evidence of the benefits of vitamin C, vitamin E, beta carotene, alpha-lipoic acid, CoQ10, N-acetyl cysteine, and selenium in preserving brain cells. These antioxidants are an integral part of our comprehensive program for the treatment of mild to moderate Alzheimer's disease. We recommend the following daily doses of antioxidant supplements:

Vitamin C	1,000 mg
Vitamin E	300 IU
Beta carotene	10,000 IU (do not take if you are a smoker or have smoked in the past ten years)
Alpha-lipoic acid	500 mg
CoQ10	100 mg by gel cap (Ubiquinol is preferred over ubiquinone. If you take a statin medication, we recommend doubling this dose.)
N-Acetyl Cysteine	1,500 mg
Selenium	200 mcg (micrograms)

If possible, these supplements should be taken with food. It is also a good idea to divide the doses in half and take them twice daily. Find a broad-spectrum antioxidant formula that provides most of these nutrients. This will reduce the number of supplement bottles on your shelf and add up to fewer pills to take each day. This is important because these are not the only supplements that you will be taking in our Six-Step Program; this group includes just the specific antioxidants we use.

We use many supplements, all with published evidence of their effectiveness in combating Alzheimer's. We combine our recommended supplements in groups to minimize the number of pills our patients must take. We also combine the majority of these in a tasty powdered drink formula called Epigenetic Symphony. (Other supplements will be described in upcoming chapters.)

Exercise

Studies have shown that regular exercise is even more powerful at reducing chronic oxidative stress than is taking antioxidant supplements. Regular exercise can reduce oxidative stress and improve cell energy production and function.

Sticking to a regular schedule of exercise sessions is ideal, but any level of activity is beneficial. Many AD patients are unable to exercise with intensity, but regular walks or other enjoyable light activity can still provide tremendous benefit and should be made a high priority.

The Science

Exercise contributes to optimal health and disease prevention in numerous ways, but one powerful result includes a dramatically enhanced capacity to deal with free radicals. Paradoxically, sessions of exercise temporarily increase the production of oxygen free radicals. This "stress" then acts as a powerful stimulus for the body to increase production of its own antioxidant molecules (glutathione, for example). Much of this process takes place in the cell's power plant, the mitochondria, and may even involve an increase in the number of mitochondria.

STEP 1: Summary of Recommendations

The recommendations in Step 1 are part of our broad-spectrum program designed to arrest or even reverse mild to moderate Alzheimer's disease. Overwhelming evidence shows that all elements and aspects of this program have a biochemical impact on the *root causes* of Alzheimer's. Step 1's recommendations have one overarching goal: to limit oxidative stress.

1. Avoid exposure to aluminum, mercury, copper, and excessive iron.

2. Measure your serum ferritin level, and donate blood if necessary to keep it below 100 ng/ml. If the blood bank won't take your blood, ask your doctor for a prescription to have phlebotomies (blood removal) performed.

3. Avoid air pollution by using the strategies and techniques we describe on page 31.

4. Drink only water treated with reverse osmosis or distillation, and supplement the following minerals: calcium, magnesium, and potassium (see page 27).

5. Eat as much organic produce as possible. Ideally, this should be your primary source of fuel.

6. Take a broad-spectrum antioxidant supplement formula. These are available in retail stores. We encourage you to consider our formula, Epigenetic Symphony, designed to provide these antioxidants along with calcium, magnesium, potassium, and additional nutrients found to combat the root causes of AD, conveniently packaged as a flavored drink mix to be taken twice a day. These two daily drinks provide nutrients that would otherwise require thirty capsules.

7. Apply phytate cream daily to your skin to help bond toxic heavy metals in the blood and brain. The recommended dose is one-quarter teaspoon of a 50 percent preparation.

8. Avoid electromagnetic fields (EMF) to the best of your ability.

9. If your physician gives you the go-ahead, exercise as vigorously and regularly as possible, preferably at least thirty minutes per day at a heart rate between 70 and 90 percent of your calculated maximum (see step 2, p. 46 for these details).

STEP 2   Prevent "Sticky" Proteins
Limit Glycation

Have you ever stepped on a piece of chewing gum? First the gum sticks to the sole of your shoe, and then with each step the gum picks up other dirt, grass, and anything else it touches. The process called glycation works in a similar way, only instead of happening with gum and the sole of your shoe, it happens in our bodies when sugar and protein stick together.

Glycation is a *normal* process that happens constantly inside all of us. Excess glycation, however, is bad for our health. Excess glycation is related to the development of virtually every age-related disease.

The faster glycation occurs, the sooner we develop a number of serious age-related diseases, including dementia. Fortunately, we can relieve our bodies of the stress of excess glycation by making wise choices with food and by exercising. But before we get to that, let's look at *why* glycation is so harmful to us.

Excess Glycation Kills Brain Cells

Proteins are large molecules that move around in our cells performing very important functions. They are our cellular engineers. There are thousands of different proteins in our cells, and each one has a different function. With thousands of these giant proteins moving around in each cell, they often bump into each other, but because they're very slippery they usually slide right off one another without causing any harm; biochemically speaking, they repel one another. Unfortunately, when we have high levels of sugar in our blood the proteins lose their slippery advantage.

Sugar, or glucose, is body and brain fuel, so we definitely need it. The trouble is that most people are getting way too much, which is a problem because glucose is naturally attracted to protein molecules. Whenever glucose and a protein collide, they stick together instead of sliding by each other. The slippery protein gets coated with this "sugar glue"—like gum on your shoe—and then it gets stuck to other proteins, making a sticky mess. Not only does this stop the proteins from doing their jobs, but it also makes more work for the trash removal crew, aka our immune system.

Scientists call these piles of protein-sugar garbage advanced glycation end products, or *AGEs* (ay-gee-eez) for short. They came up with this name because the first letters of these three words spell "AGE" and they wanted to show the association of advanced glycation end products with the aging process. (Scientists love acronyms!)

Our immune system's white blood cells dissolve the trash piles by releasing chemicals called cytokines. The problem is that cytokines are not smart bombs—they're more like shotgun fire, spraying and affecting everything in the general vicinity. Therefore, in doing their jobs, they injure other structures like our brain cells. The damage that occurs during trash removal is called inflammation. And inflammation, like glycation itself, is linked to a wide variety of chronic diseases, including, of course, Alzheimer's.

If that double whammy isn't enough to keep your hand out of the cookie jar, this next bit of information should do the trick. These sticky protein-and-sugar trash piles attach themselves to the receptors designed to find them (Receptors for AGEs[1] = RAGE). When this happens, the cell becomes a virtual war zone. All sorts of bad chemistry occurs, including the creation of large armies of free radicals, causing oxidative stress. This is very damaging to all our cells but particularly destructive to our fragile brain cells.

Each brain cell can handle only a certain amount of trash (AGEs), cytokines, and free radicals before it dies. So, the more glycation, oxidative stress, and resultant inflammation we have in our bodies and brains, the faster we lose brain cells. When we look at MRI (magnetic resonance imaging) pictures of the brain, we can see if a brain is shrinking, and if it is, we know that the person has fewer brain cells than he did before. This is a universal finding in Alzheimer's disease.

So, just like with oxidative stress in Step 1, we need to minimize the damage from glycation in Step 2.

The Science of AGEs

There are lots of studies attempting to link AGEs with the beta-amyloid plaques in people with Alzheimer's disease. In fact, AGEs have been found in higher numbers in Alzheimer's brains, and they've been found to be present in both amyloid plaques and neurofibrillary tangles—the two abnormal structures that form in Alzheimer's brains. It's not clear whether AGEs actually promote the beta-amyloid protein or the neurofibrillary tangles. What is clear is that whether or not they contribute directly to the formation of the plaques or tangles, they absolutely join with the plaques and tangles to kill brain cells.

High Blood Sugar

We have total control over the glucose level in our blood because in order for glucose to get to our blood, we have to put it into our mouths. The lower our blood sugar, the less we glycate and the more brain cells we save. Now, we're not talking about *unnaturally* low blood sugar, but optimal blood sugar. Optimal blood sugar level when first waking in the morning is between 55 and 90 mg/dl. Optimally, blood sugar should peak no higher than 130 mg/dl *or less* 60 to 90 minutes after a meal or snack but otherwise should remain below 115 mg/dl for the remainder of the day.

Because of modern food processing and inactive lifestyles, nearly every person in the United States has blood-sugar levels that are above optimal much of the day. We may think of this as "normal," since we're used to carbo-loading and sugarcoating our food, but trust us—it is *not* natural. And it is not healthy.

The Science of High Blood Sugar

Every time we raise our blood sugar, our body has to process that extra glucose. Processing requires the hormone called insulin. The higher we raise our blood sugar, the more insulin we must make, because insulin escorts the sugar into our cells to be burned for energy. If our cells get an excess of energy, it's stored as fat.

Repeatedly raising blood sugar above optimal levels results in excess body fat. In turn, excess fat makes it harder for insulin to process sugar, a condition called insulin resistance. Our bodies compensate for insulin resistance by making more insulin. Unfortunately, this results in more fat storage, which leads to more insulin resistance. This is the perpetual cycle that leads to obesity and type II diabetes.

Insulin resistance also reduces the amount of energy available to brain cells and causes them to function poorly. Poorly functioning brain cells mean a poorly functioning brain. Moreover, the elevated insulin level caused by insulin resistance actually increases beta-amyloid production in the brain.[2] High blood sugar, then, affects multiple pathways that accelerate cognitive impairment and dramatically increase the risk for dementia. Some researchers have even referred to AD as "type III diabetes."

Keep Blood Sugar Low with Low-Glycemic Nutrition

We begin the healing process by keeping blood sugar low. Most people have a very poor understanding of how to keep blood sugar low, leading to serious dietary mistakes and a greater risk of developing all the age-related degenerative diseases, including Alzheimer's disease.

To keep blood sugar low, eat a low-glycemic diet. This will keep your blood sugar within optimal ranges and stop it from spiking into the brain-destructive high range throughout the day.

The Basics of Low Glycemic Nutrition

1. There are only three foods on the planet:
   a. Proteins (meat, fish, eggs, dairy)
   b. Fats (nuts, seeds, oils)
   c. Carbohydrates, or carbs (fruits, nonstarch vegetables, sweets, starches)

2. Of these three, only carbohydrates significantly raise blood sugar. But not all carbs are created equal. It's best to forget the older terms *simple carbs* and *complex carbs* and instead use *low glycemic* (nonstarch vegetables) and *high glycemic* (sweets and starches). Fruits are an intermediate category.

3. Avoid sweets and starches because they are high glycemic and raise blood sugar more than other carbohydrates. This is true regardless of whether you consider them simple or complex carbs or whether they are white or brown.

4. Eat all the nonstarch vegetables you'd like, because they don't raise blood sugar.

5. Eat fruit in moderation and limit servings (one piece = one serving) to no more than four per day.

Avoid Sweets and Starches

There's a lot of confusion about what is considered a sweet and what is considered a starch, so we're going to make this as simple as possible.

Sweets are carbohydrates containing sugar that taste sweet. These include candy, pastry, baked goods, soda pop, fruit juice (soda pop with vitamins), sweetened dairy products like flavored yogurt and ice cream, and virtually everything that might appear on a dessert menu. (Realistically, everyone is going to have a little something sweet now and then. In these instances, these artificial sweeteners, while not ideal, are certainly better than sugar: sucralose (Splenda), xylitol (a sugar alcohol), and stevia, a sugar substitute made from a leaf that happens to taste very sweet. We do *not* recommend saccharin or aspartame as sweeteners.

Starches include potatoes, peas, and all foods made from wheat, rice, corn, oats, rye, barley, quinoa, millet, amaranth, and other grains. For those of you in denial, these include bread, cereal, chips, crackers, and all baked goods made from grains. It doesn't matter what color they are or whether they're sweet—starches will spike your blood sugar because they are high glycemic.

Now that you have these simple concepts committed to memory, there are a few exceptions. (Aren't there always?)

Six Acceptable Starches in Limited Serving Sizes

1. Oatmeal limited to three to four ounces by dry volume per serving. Do not use instant; use rolled oats or steel-cut oats. After cooking, add a heaping tablespoon of organic almond or peanut butter and a scoop of whey protein to further diminish impact on blood sugar (and provide more of a meal).

2. A small bowl (four ounces or less) of 100 percent bran cereal (unsweetened).

3. Brown rice, in a side-dish portion eaten with other foods as part of a meal.

4. Pasta, in a side-dish portion (not as an entrée).

5. Beans, in a side-dish portion.

6. Split-kernel and bran breads. Be *very* careful here: Some of the very chewy and chunky breads may be acceptable, but do your research first.

For more information and comprehensive lists of the glycemic characteristics of numerous foods, see www.glycemicindex.com or www.mendosa.com. While we can't verify the accuracy of information on these sites, we have found them to be accurate and up to date over the years.

Three Tricks to Further Reduce the Glycemic Load of Any Carbohydrate

1. Add protein: lean meats, nuts, protein supplement

2. Add fiber: vegetables, berries, fiber supplement

3. Add "good" fat: nuts and nut butters, olive oil, avocado

These three components slow your digestion, and, therefore, your absorption of sugar. Keep in mind, however, that even though mixing protein, fiber, or fat in with carbs will reduce the amount of glycation, serving sizes must still be kept small.

Where Does Fruit Fit In?

Fruits are carbohydrates, but they also contain antioxidants, so you definitely want to keep eating most types of fruit. The keys here are to avoid fruits that are high on the glycemic index and to limit yourself to one piece or serving of fruit per meal. Eating more than that will spike your blood sugar just as much as a large bowl of pasta or rice. The following fruits are high glycemic and should be avoided:

▶ Bananas

▶ Kiwi

▶ Mangoes

▶ Papaya

▶ Watermelon

Fruit Juice

You should also avoid fruit juice, and this is true whether it comes from the store or you make it yourself. One serving of fruit juice contains the sugar from several pieces of fruit. And because it typically has no pulp (fiber), it digests rapidly and spikes your blood sugar just like a glass of soda pop. One exception is tomato juice, but be sure to limit the amount to eight ounces per serving.

High-Glycemic Vegetables and Vegetable Juices

High-glycemic vegetables should also be avoided; these include beets and peas. Beet juice and carrot juice are not recommended, but carrots as a side dish are fine due to their fiber content.

Aside from beet and carrot juices, other vegetable juices are fine, particularly those made from greens like kale and spinach. But to keep your blood sugar low, liquefying whole vegetables in the blender is preferable to juicing. This is because blending the veggies keeps the fiber in your drink, whereas juicing them does not.

The Bottom Line on Carbohydrates

Ideally, most of your carbs should come from *nonstarch vegetables.*

What to Embrace

Exercise

Exercise immediately reduces blood sugar and promotes good blood-sugar control. This effect on blood sugar is one of the mechanisms by which exercise has been shown in clinical studies to reduce the risk of AD as well as substantially benefit AD patients.[4-8] But there are also others.

The Science of Exercise

As we discussed in Step 1, exercise creates oxygen free radicals (oxidative stress), and the body compensates for this by producing more antioxidants. The overall effect from exercise-induced oxidative stress and the resultant production of antioxidants is extremely healthy.

In addition, exercising puts our bodies in a healthy defensive mode. This defensive mode makes our bodies produce proteins (cellular engineers) that are protective to our brains.

Two of these protective proteins are called heat-shock protein[9] and brain-derived neurotrophic factor (BDNF).[10] These proteins protect brain cells in general, and they also protect them specifically from the toxicity of beta-amyloid protein.

Not only that, but the protein called BDNF actually help us to *grow new brain cells!* That's right—researchers have discovered that we can continually grow new brain cells.

Exercise also helps keep us stronger and more flexible, and it improves our mood, which is very important to quality of life for everyone, but particularly for people with Alzheimer's disease.

What Kind? How Much? How Often?

These are the top three questions our patients ask when we fill them in on all the amazing benefits of exercise. Ideally, your exercise routine will include aerobic training, strength training, and flexibility (what we used to call stretching).

Of course, see your doctor for an evaluation before you begin an exercise program to determine if it's safe, and always listen to your body.

Aerobic Training

For people with Alzheimer's disease, the most important type of exercise is aerobic training. Aerobic training includes bicycling (stationary or outdoors), jogging (treadmill, elliptical machine or outdoors), stair climbing, swimming, and any steady activity that increases your heart rate.

Walking is okay if you honestly can't do anything else. But if you're walking instead of doing a more strenuous workout simply because you don't like physical exertion or you feel lazy, you need to take it up a notch. Find a workout partner or a fitness coach to help you create and maintain an exercise program that is most appropriate for your abilities and needs.

If you have joint problems, find a place to swim or see if you can bicycle or use the elliptical trainer or stair climber.

In general, you should raise your heart rate to between 70 and 90 percent of your calculated maximum heart rate. For those who are fit and without cardiovascular disease or who have been cleared by a physician for high-intensity exercise, exceeding 90 percent of your maximum heart rate can provide additional health benefits. High-intensity exercise requires recovery periods of low-intensity activity for maximum benefit. Your calculated maximum heart rate is roughly 220 minus your age. For example: if you're 63 years old, your calculated maximum heart rate is 157 (220 − 63). You would then exercise with a sustained heart rate between 110 (70% of 157) and 141 (90% of 157).

Ideally, you should incorporate aerobic exercise seven days a week and for at least thirty and preferably sixty minutes a day. If you find this impossible, come as close as you can to the recommendation. Your benefit will be proportional to your level of participation.

Strength or Resistance Training

Strength training includes lifting weights and doing exercises like push-ups, sit-ups, and pull-ups that increase your strength, but it improves more than strength. Strength training also improves bone density, helping to prevent fragility fractures (typically of the hips, wrists, and spine). This can be instrumental in preventing serious setbacks in progress against Alzheimer's disease and in health in general. Mix strength training into your workout three to five times a week.

If you have limitations, do whatever you possibly can. Be creative in working around disabilities. One study showed that even a short walk outdoors was able to improve performance on a memory test, so every little movement helps. A well-educated personal trainer can be instrumental in helping to customize a program to an individual's limitations.

Flexibility

As we grow older, our muscles tend to get tighter. To maintain flexibility and avoid putting excess stress on our joints, we need to include stretching in our exercise routines. This can be as unstructured as bending and stretching whatever feels tight or would benefit from being looser. Or it can be a more structured routine like following along with a yoga tape or attending a class.

The bottom line here is that exercise is extremely beneficial in treating AD, in preventing AD, and in slowing aging in general. *NOTE TO CARETAKERS:* Strongly encourage your Alzheimer's patients to exercise, and participate with them if necessary. Whatever they can do, get them moving to the best of their ability.

STEP 2: Summary of Recommendations

Remember that each part of our broad-spectrum program designed to arrest or reverse mild to moderate Alzheimer's disease is very important for the success of the overall program. Every recommendation we make is based on scientific evidence. The theme of the recommendations of Step 2 is Limit Glycation:

1. Remove sweets and starches from your diet. Having a "treat" once a week or so is okay, but remember that it will take its toll.

2. Avoid watermelon, bananas, kiwi, papaya, mangoes, and all fruit juices.

3. Avoid peas, beets, and juices made from beets and carrots.

4. Get your carbohydrates as *completely* as possible from nonstarch vegetables and from limited-size servings of the six acceptable starches (p. 42).

5. Exercise every day for thirty minutes to an hour. Your exercise should include aerobics, strength training and flexibility (stretching).

Step 3   Make Your Genes Work in Your Favor
The Magic of the Multisupplement

U p until about twenty years ago, it was universally believed that our health, disease risk, and death were determined entirely by our genes. The genetic blueprint we inherited from our parents was believed to be our destiny, and, at least in theory, no matter what we did or didn't do, we could be doomed from the start.

Fortunately, this old belief has proved to be false in a big way. We are not at the mercy of our genes; they can be turned on and off by the choices we make in our everyday lives. And one of the most important choices we can make is to supplement our diets with a nutritional supplement formula designed to switch on the "good" genes and switch off the "bad."

We know this because over the past two decades enormous progress has been made in biological science. The sciences of epigenetics and proteomics, in particular, are providing us with astonishing and very encouraging proof that our genetic blueprint is only *one* factor in determining the fate of our health. It turns out that we have far more control than we ever thought possible!

The Science of Our Genes

Scientists have learned that our genetic blueprint is much like a set of light switches, meaning that our genes can be turned on or turned off—expressed or not expressed. Our genes affect our health because they manufacture proteins that operate all of our bodies' chemical reactions.

We have millions of different proteins in our bodies working together or competing with each other in millions of ways. Some combinations of proteins are good for health, reducing disease risk, and others are bad, increasing disease risk.

▶ If genes for a harmful combination of proteins are expressed (turned on), it increases our risk for disease.

▶ If these harmful combinations are turned off, our disease risk is reduced.

And it works the opposite way for healthy combinations of proteins:

▶ When these healthy combinations of proteins are turned on, we reduce our disease risk.

▶ When they're turned off, we increase our risk.

The operation of our gene switches—our epigenetics—is arguably more influential than our genetic blueprint in determining if and when we contract a degenerative disease. By operating the switches, we have stronger input on which proteins are being made and not made.

The science of proteomics is an extension of epigenetics. Proteomics studies how those millions of proteins ordered up by our genes interact. The complexity is as overwhelming as the workings of the universe. Although proteomics is still in its infancy, it has already contributed volumes to our understanding of prevention and reversal of Alzheimer's and other diseases.

How to Control the Switchboard

Our goal is to keep our healthy genes switched on and our harmful genes switched off. Our challenge—and our opportunity—is that just about everything we do affects our epigenetic switching.

The air we breathe, the food we eat, the water and other beverages we drink, our physical and mental activities, and the chemicals we're exposed to all have a hand in flipping our gene switches on or off. That means that almost every decision we make changes our gene expression in some way. Our nutrition, behavior, and environmental exposure determine which gene combinations (both protective and destructive) turn on and which turn off.

Nutrients, in particular, are powerful determinants of our epigenetics. This is confirmed by animal studies and human clinical trials. Scientific literature includes thousands of illustrations of how nutritional compounds affect gene expression. So there is no question that our nutrition plays a major role in turning our switches on and off.

Some of the most profound results were demonstrated through a series of studies conducted by Drs. Lemon, Boreham, and Rollo and colleagues at McMaster University in Ontario, Canada.[1-5] Rather than looking at one nutritional supplement in isolation, the traditional type of study, these researchers took a leap of faith and decided to study a large set of supplements as a group. Each supplement they included had been shown to produce some benefit in the areas of reducing oxidative stress, glycation, and inflammation. Although not one of these supplements by itself had a profound, life-altering effect, the research team theorized that combining these beneficial supplements could produce better results.

The upside in this type of study is that there is a greater likelihood that combining beneficial supplements, rather than administering them individually, will have a profound effect. The downside is that if it does, we won't know which of the ingredients was most influential.

To this, Lemon, Boreham, and Rollo said, "So what?".

Being results-oriented, they plunged forward using the whole enchilada—some twenty-eight ingredients in all. They chose the ingredients based on benefits that had been demonstrated in previous studies. Each ingredient had one or more of the following beneficial properties:

1. Antioxidant

2. Antiglycating (by helping to control blood sugar)

3. Anti-inflammatory

4. Supportive of the membrane function of either the cell itself or the mitochondria—the energy factories within the cells

Sounds Great! But Does It Work?

Next, the research team tested this multinutrient formula on mice. Why mice? For three reasons: First, mice have a genetic makeup that overlaps with ours by about 98 percent. Second, mice live only about thirty months, allowing us to study a lifelong health profile in about 3 percent of the time it would take to study the same profile in humans. Finally, these mice lived in a laboratory environment so that every activity and every molecule that entered their mouths could be controlled, allowing for a completely scientific comparison between groups. (Try that with humans!).

Mice were started on this nutritional formula immediately after being weaned and continued on it for their entire lives. The formula was added to their food at a very precise dose. These mice were compared with a control group that was fed the same food but was not given the supplement formula. The living conditions for the two groups were identical, as was the genetic lineage. The *only* difference between the groups was the formula itself.

The study found that when the mice on the formula reached old age, they were cognitively superior and more physically active than the *young* adult mice that were not receiving the formula! These results are nothing less than astounding.

When we read this study, our first thought was, "That's the multi for us and our patients!"

The mice receiving the multi formula also lived 11 percent longer as a group. This nutritional formula had a profound epigenetic effect in terms of disease prevention, cognitive function, strength, physical mobility, and life extension.

This series of studies has enormous implications in preventing, arresting, or reversing AD. Even if the evidence were limited to the McMaster University studies, we would be optimistic, but the evidence is far more extensive than just these animal studies. Many of the ingredients in the McMaster formulation had been individually tested previously in test-tube, animal, and human clinical trials and showed substantial promise. Many of these studies were conducted among humans with Alzheimer's disease and animals bred to develop AD. We'll look at each of these ingredients and their related studies in Step 4.

Keep in mind, though, that while nutrients and supplements are a big part of our program, so are lifestyle and the all-important hormone replacement that we'll cover in Step 5.

Each ingredient used in the McMaster studies has been used in humans very safely, so we converted the mouse dose into the human dose and assembled all the ingredients from the study that could be combined into a single powdered formula. To this we added a few more ingredients that, from our research, proved to be of additional benefit. We call this formula Epigenetic Symphony, for obvious reasons: the ingredients work together like the instruments in a symphony orchestra to more effectively optimize our gene expression (boost the function of protective genes and suppress the destructive ones) all to engineer peak performance (both physical and mental) and the ultimate in disease protection.

Epigenetic Symphony forms the base of our nutritional supplement protocol for both our Optimal Health Programs and our Alzheimer's Program. The ingredients from the McMaster University studies that could not be combined into our powdered formula are available in capsules (at www.Cycle-Breakers.com). In Step 4, we'll list all the ingredients and discuss which aspects of disease protection they engineer and how that applies to Alzheimer's disease. All the supplements we use for AD have benefit in terms of epigenetics or proteomics or both. For now, we want to cover the components of Epigenetic Symphony that are very important for overall health.

The nutrients in Table 3.1 are components of a good multimineral, multivitamin formula. They each have specific functions that are beneficial in the prevention of diseases, but keep in mind that each was part of that *multi-ingredient formula* that preserved (and improved) youthful cognitive and physical function in mice. Also remember that just because we can't describe the formula's mechanistic pathway in regard to AD doesn't mean the specific *combination* of components isn't crucial to getting the full benefits.

Table 3.1 Ingredients in Epigenetic Symphony derived from the McMaster University studies that are important for general health.

Nutrient	General Health Benefit
Vitamin B1 (Thiamine): 50 mg	Energy production from food
Vitamin B2 (Riboflavin): 25 mg	Energy production from food
Vitamin B3: (Niacin) 50 mg	Energy production from food
Vitamin K: 0.5 mg	Necessary for normal blood clotting and for strong bones
Boron: 0.75 mg	Preserves bone density by retaining calcium and activating vitamin D and estrogen
Bromelain: 30 mg	Digestive enzyme; aids in extracting nutrients from foods
Broccoli extract: 100 mg	Cancer prevention (glucosinolates → indoles)
Calcium: 800 mg	Benefits virtually every human organ system
Copper: 0.2 mg	Component of many essential enzymes
L-Glutathione: 72 mg	Important antioxidant but, when taken orally, probably benefits only the intestinal cells
Magnesium: 100 mg	More than three hundred functions in the human body
Potassium: 72 mg	A key mineral electrolyte involved in much of normal body chemistry
Horsetail extract (silica): 0.7 mg	An important mineral for bone density
Diindolylmethane (DIM): 100 mg	Indole compound for cancer prevention

STEP 3: Summary of Recommendations

Take a good, broad spectrum multivitamin, multimineral, antioxidant and anti-glycating nutritional supplement. The table above lists those important for general health. Further details on exactly what to take are provided in Step 4: Summary of Recommendations. In the steps that follow, we'll cover all the components of Epigenetic Symphony and our other key supplements that have specific activity against Alzheimer's and include a description of how they work. Keep in mind that just as the combination of nutrients in the McMaster study improved the results, the combination of all the components in our program is necessary for producing the best possible results. Nutritional supplements are just one of the important integrative components of our program.

STEP 4   Combat the Root Causes of Alzheimer's Disease
Protect and Defend Your Brain

To effectively treat AD, we must use a comprehensive, integrated approach. Since dementia is the end result of numerous destructive processes that occur over time, targeting just one or two of these processes won't cut it. We have to address the long list of biochemical and physiological events that influence the destruction.

We do this by giving our bodies the support they need to head off these destructive processes and heal from the ones already underway. As we said in the introduction, there is no magic bullet that can prevent or reverse AD, because there are too many root causes for just one form of treatment or prevention.

That's why we must do our preventive and healing work at the "ecological level." Our ecology is determined by the way we approach the world around us; it is largely in our control because it is all about our lifestyle and the choices we make each day. At this level, we can exert powerful, healing influence and significantly alter the course and speed of AD. The key to success is an integrated comprehensive health plan.

Integration is also important when it comes to using supplements. Taking a variety of supplements can provide measurable benefits, including the relief of some symptoms, but it won't be enough to alter the outcome of the disease. To change the future, we must use the *right combination* of supplements in the *correct dosages*, in the context of a comprehensive treatment plan.

The great news is that the supplements in the plan we recommend are supported by evidence that shows that they can be effective in preventing and treating AD.

Why We Chose These Supplements

A Brief Review of the Key Fundamental Processes in AD

The hallmark abnormalities in AD are the accumulation of beta-amyloid plaque and neurofibrillary tangles (NFTs) in the brain. In healthy brains, a significant accumulation of plaque does not occur.

This plaque is formed from a specific protein called amyloid precursor protein (APP). But the protein doesn't do the manufacturing on its own. It relies on the actions of two main enzymes: one is called beta secretase, and the other is gamma secretase.

What's great is that *other* enzymes can turn APP into a harmless protein. The activity of these enzymes, both the harmful and harmless, can be influenced and modified by many of the components discussed throughout this book, including supplements. Our goal is to stimulate enzymes that turn APP into the harmless protein and inhibit those that promote beta-amyloid protein.

Just as important as reducing plaque accumulation is the removal of plaque that is already present. The plaque (beta amyloid) is cleared by immune cells in the brain called microglia (my-crow-glee-uh). We can also stimulate the microglia to speed up the process of clearing beta amyloid from the brain.

You recall that the other culprit in AD is the structure called neurofibrillary tangles (NFTs). We don't yet fully understand the mechanisms that form NFTs, but we do know that a process that activates or deactivates many protein enzymes is involved. This process, called *phosphorylation* (fos-for-ill-ation), is also influenced by many factors, including certain supplements. An important protein in our brain cells called *tau* is responsible for the structural integrity of the brain cell much like a steel frame supports a building. In AD the tau protein undergoes too much of this phosphorylation process, resulting in structural changes called crosslinking and cleavage. The crosslinking and cleavage, in turn, cause the tau protein to flex in the wrong places and actually curl up to form useless *tangles* in brain cells. The brain cell then loses its structural integrity. An analogy would be the melting of a building's steel frame. When brain cells lose their structural integrity they can't survive. This is how tau, along with excessive beta amyloid protein, kills brain cells in AD. Below are diagrams that summarize the processes behind beta amyloid accumulation and the formation of NFTs. As you read about the supplements you can refer back to these diagrams.

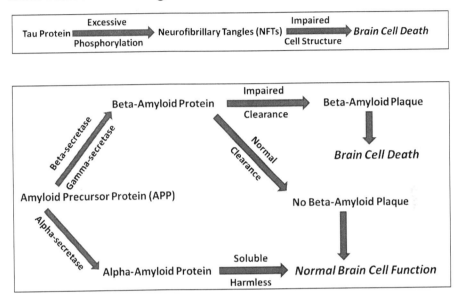

So, to a significant extent, we can influence the two prominent instigators of Alzheimer's disease in three ways:

1. Producing less beta-amyloid protein

2. Clearing beta-amyloid plaque that's already present

3. Producing fewer neurofibrillary tangles

But remember, the way the plaques and tangles cause trouble is by being toxic to brain cells and literally killing them. So there is yet another way we can positively influence Alzheimer's: by protecting our brain cells from the toxicity of the plaques and tangles, allowing them to function and survive in the presence of these abnormal proteins. Protecting our brain cells from plaques and tangles is accomplished first by reducing oxidation and glycation, which we covered in Steps 1 and 2. This, in turn will reduce inflammation and improve insulin sensitivity, cell signaling, cell receptor function, and energy production (mitochondrial function). Please don't worry about memorizing these processes. We will reduce all this to a list of *do*s and *don't*s. We just want you to recognize that our program is based on the best available biochemistry on Alzheimer's. In addition to nutrition, exercise, sleep, stress, hormones, and environmental factors, there are many supplements known to affect these variables.

Strengthening Our Front Lines of Defense

The following supplements tip the scales in favor of preventing and reversing Alzheimer's disease. If you're anything like our patients, finding out how supplements combat the root causes of AD will probably make you happy to take them. Don't be put off by the names—what's important is that each one is a powerful weapon in your arsenal against AD.

Also, as you read about each of these effective supplements and the study results, you may have a tendency to think that each is helpful but not a cure. You're right! But remember, we're betting that the combination, never tried before in history, will swing the pendulum of Alzheimer's the other way.

Acetyl-L-Carnitine (ALCAR)

ALCAR has been researched in human subjects for some time, and several studies have shown it to be beneficial in preventing cognitive impairment and dementia. In fact, no fewer than seven double-blind placebo-controlled human trials of ALCAR in AD patients, using from 1.2 to 3 grams daily, have shown that this supplement may slow the decline in or improve performance on cognitive function tests. In several of these studies, the benefit of this supplement was limited to patients with early-onset AD (fifty- to seventy-year-olds).[1–7]

The preliminary evidence of benefit in small human trials and the excellent safety profile of this supplement warrant its use in the prevention and treatment of AD. This position is further reinforced by more recent studies in animal models of AD showing that AL-CAR inhibits several key pathways in the development of AD, including oxidative damage, the production of beta-amyloid protein, the cleavage of tau protein, apoptosis (cell self-destruction), and cellular stress intolerance.[8-15] *This single supplement operates on four of our nine avenues.*

Alpha-Lipoic Acid (LA)

Alpha-lipoic acid may actually slow or prevent progression of AD. In 2001, a study was published with the title "Alpha-lipoic acid as a new treatment option for Alzheimer type dementia."[16] Although this study was small (nine AD patients), it showed stabilization of the patients' cognitive function over eleven months, suggesting that LA, at a dose of 600 mg daily, may be useful in preventing progression of the disease. In 2007, the same group published the results of a study that was larger (forty-eight patients) and longer (two years). This study showed that AD progressed very slowly in the LA group, compared with a much more rapid progression in the conventional-treatment group (receiving the standard FDA-approved anticholinesterase drugs).[17] These small studies demonstrated that LA was far superior to the commonly prescribed but mostly ineffective conventional treatments, and the authors pleaded for more clinical trials using LA. Unfortunately, no trials followed, since clinical trials are expensive and LA, like all supplements, is not patentable and therefore not profitable enough for a drug company to spend millions to prove its efficacy to the FDA. Small groups of researchers continued their work on LA in hopes of persuading the medical community to adopt this compound. Their research showed that LA inhibits oxidation and the cellular toxicity of beta amyloid, increases levels of the natural antioxidant glutathione, improves mitochondrial energy production, increases mitochondrial number, and improves insulin sensitivity. All these mechanisms help brain cells to remain vital and functional in the face of attack. In animal models of AD, LA has consistently demonstrated the ability to dramatically slow progression of dementia. Common doses were often near a human equivalent of 1400 mg daily.[18–21] *LA works along at least four of our nine avenues.*

Vitamins B3, B6, and B12

The benefits of certain B vitamins to the brain are several, but the most important benefit is in the control of *homocysteine.* Homocysteine is an amino acid (component of proteins) that we all have in our body. Our level of homocysteine can easily be measured by a blood test, and the normal range defined at most laboratories is 5 to 11 umol/L. At the Leonardi Institute, our motto is that *normal* is not necessarily *optimal.* Higher levels of homocysteine have long been associated with risk of AD. Below we'll cite for you a study demonstrating that the risk of AD increases by 50 percent for every 5 umol/L rise in the homocysteine level.[34] Therefore, if your homocysteine level is 10 and your doctor calls it normal, he or she is correct—but he or she may not inform you that your risk of AD is 50 percent higher than that of someone whose level is 5. In our evaluations of new patients, we find a wide range of homocysteine levels and many are above 14 umol/L, a level associated with *double* the risk of AD. Homocysteine is processed and removed from the body by a series of chemical reactions mostly dependent on specific nutrients: vitamins B6 and B12, folic acid, and trimethylglycine (TMG). Another important nutrient, N-acetyl cysteine (NAC), binds homocysteine and carries it out through the kidneys via the urine. At the Leonardi Institute, we measure and reduce homocysteine levels regularly using these nutrients. We often find that fairly high doses are required to reduce homocysteine into the *lower end* of the normal range. Homocysteine control is not the only feature, but a major one as we introduce the B vitamins that support brain cells.

B vitamins, specifically vitamins B6 and B12, promote cognitive and neurological function, lower homocysteine levels, and protect brain cells from homocysteine toxicity.

There is substantial evidence that low levels of vitamins B6, B12, and folic acid are associated with higher levels of homocysteine and that higher levels of homocysteine participate in the destruction of brain cells underlying AD.

Vitamin B3 (nicotinamide) has a number of remarkable effects targeting the root causes of Alzheimer's disease. These are discussed in detail on the next page.

B vitamins are critical cofactors in numerous biochemical reactions and enzymatic pathways, leading to their elevated status among the general public as health and energy-generating supplements. Additionally, deficiencies in certain B vitamins are known to cause cognitive and neurological dysfunction, such as in "megaloblastic madness" and Wernike-Korsakoff syndrome.

At the same time, homocysteine levels increase when we have inadequate levels of the B vitamins folate, B12, and B6. Supplementing these vitamins is an effective way to lower homocysteine levels. Researchers examining homocysteine and B-vitamin levels in AD patients discovered that Alzheimer's victims had both elevated homocysteine levels and reduced levels of folate and B12, compared with healthy controls.[25] Subsequent research demonstrated that elevated homocysteine levels precede the development of AD and are therefore a significant risk factor for the disease as well as for vascular dementia and stroke.[26,27] A more recent study examined the relationship between vitamin B12, homocysteine, and risk for AD and found, again, that both low B12 levels and high homocysteine levels were associated with the development of dementia.[28] Furthermore, using sophisticated statistical analysis, this study was able to demonstrate that elevated homocysteine and its association with AD is at least partly explained by the inadequate B12 levels. These epidemiologic studies convincingly established homocysteine and low B-vitamin levels as risk factors for AD, but the mechanisms behind these associations remained unclear. However, evidence is now accumulating that elevated homocysteine and low B-vitamin levels can exacerbate cellular vulnerability to the oxidative damage and brain-cell death induced by beta-amyloid plaque.[29,30]

A few limited trials of B-vitamin supplementation have been conducted, with some showing benefit from supplementation and the lowering of homocysteine levels while others demonstrated little or no benefit. However, all these studies were short (two years or less), and homocysteine was only moderately lowered and/or B-vitamin status was seldom measured.[31–33]

Finally, an article published July 2011 in *Alzheimer's and Dementia: The Journal of the Alzheimer's Association* combined and analyzed the results of eight previous studies involving 8,669 participants. It showed that for every five-micromole-per-liter increase in the blood level of homocysteine, there was a 50 percent increase in Alzheimer's risk. Clearly, it's important to control homocysteine to prevent AD and even more important for those who have AD.[34]

In our program, one goal is to keep serum levels of homocysteine below 7 mg/L (milligrams per liter), despite the fact that levels up to 11 are considered normal-once again, normal is not necessarily optimal. To do this, we use a combination of vitamins B6 and B12 along with folic acid and trimethylglycine in the optimal dose combination. We call this formula Homocysteine Processor. Specialty formulas like Homocysteine Processor simplify the task of taking multiple nutritional supplements in the optimal dose for a specific purpose.

Nicotinamide (also called niacinamide) is one of three forms of vitamin B3 (along with niacin and nicotinic acid). Nicotinamide deserves special mention among the B vitamins due to its unique mechanisms of action against AD. While nicotinamide is involved in the relationship between homocysteine and dementia, its mechanism appears to be protecting the brain cells from homocysteine toxicity rather than lowering homocysteine.[35]

Nicotinamide's ability to protect brain cells from homocysteine and other toxins appears to involve numerous complex mechanisms. Nicotinamide has been shown to exert antioxidant, anti-inflammatory, and antiapoptotic (cellular anti-self-destruction) effects. Further, nicotinamide can improve cellular energy balance, mitochondrial function, and glucose utilization in cells under stress.[22–24] Finally, a 2008 study showed that nicotinamide reduces the phosphorylation of tau protein, which leads to neurofibrillary tangles (NFTs). In this study, mice bred to develop AD were prevented from developing multidomain cognitive impairment with daily 200 mg/kg doses of nicotinamide.[36] The human-equivalent dose of nicotinamide used in this study for a 70 kg person would be about 1,400 mg daily. However, as with every other drug or supplement studied in isolation, no benefit was observed for mice treated with nicotinamide after severe dementia was already established. This suggests that nicotinamide's greatest value might be in prevention or as a treatment when combined with other elements. *Nicotinamide acts along five of our nine avenues.*

Caffeine/Coffee

The caffeine in coffee may reduce the incidence of AD, Parkinson's disease, liver cirrhosis, and type II diabetes. It may also prevent and reverse cognitive impairment. Caffeine reduces beta-amyloid production, appears to inhibit pathways that lead to tau phosphorylation (which produces NFTs), and exerts anti-inflammatory and antioxidant activity in the brain.

Caffeine continues to receive growing attention from medical researchers after studies have shown that regular intake may reduce the incidence of type II diabetes, Parkinson's disease, and liver cirrhosis. Epidemiologic evidence has also suggested an association between coffee or caffeine consumption and a reduced risk of developing AD. For example, middle-aged people who drank three to five cups of coffee (totaling about 300 to 500 mg of caffeine) each day had a 65 percent lower risk of developing AD later in life than those who did not drink coffee.[37] Another study examined total caffeine intake over a twenty-year period and revealed that those with AD had consumed 74 mg of caffeine on average each day, while those without AD had consumed 199 mg of caffeine on average each day. *The calculated risk for developing AD was 60 percent lower for those consuming the most caffeine.*[38] In yet another study, transgenic mice that were bred to develop AD were given the human equivalent of 500 mg of caffeine (or five cups of coffee) each day. They performed as well as healthy non-transgenic mice—the expected cognitive impairment was completely prevented. Further, the mice given caffeine demonstrated significantly less beta amyloid in the hippocampus (the brain area related to memory) and reductions in beta- and gamma-secretase activity compared to transgenic controls (not receiving caffeine).[39] In another study, these same mice were not given caffeine until after they developed AD and showed marked cognitive impairment. The human equivalent of 500 mg of caffeine each day given to these AD-afflicted mice resulted in a *reversal* of their cognitive impairment and significant *reductions* in beta-amyloid levels in the brain. The study authors explained that, in addition to reducing beta-amyloid production through suppressing beta- and gamma-secretase activity, caffeine appears to inhibit pathways that lead to tau phosphorylation (which produces NFTs) and exerts anti-inflammatory and antioxidant activity in the brain.[40] Follow-up studies by the same group of researchers revealed that these effects were indeed produced by caffeine and not theophylline, a metabolite of caffeine.[41] Several studies have demonstrated that caffeine has a protective effect against the more general problem of cognitive impairment seen in normal brain aging as well.[42–44]

In the July 2011 issue of the *Journal of Alzheimer's Disease,* a research team reported a remarkable study about caffeine and coffee for Alzheimer's. The authors pointed out previous studies showing how caffeine inhibited beta-amyloid protein formation in the brain by inhibiting the activity of those two harmful enzymes, beta and gamma secretase. In this study, though, the scientists found that real coffee had additional benefits that were unobtainable from caffeine alone. They found that caffeinated coffee, but not caffeine or decaf coffee, increased the production of an important protein called granulocyte colony stimulating factor (GCSF).

GCSF is critically important because it stimulates microglia, those immune cells that clear beta-amyloid protein from the brain, to emerge from the bone marrow and do their thing. Furthermore, the authors point out previous research showing that long-term treatment with coffee (but not decaffeinated coffee) enhanced working memory in a manner associated with increased GCSF levels in the blood. The authors conclude that there must be a synergistic effect between the caffeine and another component of coffee to produce this remarkable combination of effects on Alzheimer's pathology. For this reason, at the Leonardi Institute we highly recommend daily coffee and not caffeine supplements or decaf coffee for the prevention and treatment of Alzheimer's disease.[41]

Coffee intake as a preventive or therapeutic intervention for AD should be individualized. Tolerances and side effects (such as jitteriness, anxiety, heart palpitations, and insomnia) may vary due to genetically determined enzyme activity and one's current level of daily intake. Many people are already consuming the lower evidence-supported dose of 300 mg of caffeine from coffee daily. It is not clear whether 500 mg daily will provide greater benefit, as studies comparing multiple doses have not been conducted. However, the impressive effects seen in the transgenic-mouse studies were produced by the higher dose of 500 mg per day. Tolerating this dose may require slowly increasing intake and limiting intake to the morning while abstaining from coffee after noon to prevent insomnia. If you're experiencing difficulty sleeping, this adjustment may be counterproductive, so regulate accordingly. A cup of average-strength coffee provides 100 mg of caffeine. However, specialty coffees can have a much higher caffeine content. For example, a 20-ounce (venti) house coffee at Starbucks may contain the full dose of 500 mg of caffeine.[45]

The cultivation of coffee is generally a pesticide-heavy endeavor. Therefore, choose certified organic coffee to reduce pesticide ingestion and environmental contamination. We also support choosing local or fair-trade coffee beans and grinding them just before brewing to preserve coffee's numerous phytonutrients. In summary, impressive data support coffee as a preventive and even a treatment for Alzheimer's disease. *Coffee covers at least four and possibly five of our nine avenues.*

Curcumin

Curcumin is the compound that gives the spice turmeric its yellow color. Turmeric serves as a key spice in Indian curry but is less familiar to Westerners. When it was observed that the incidence of AD in India was about four times less than that in the United States, researchers speculated that curcumin could be involved.[46] Curcumin is a very powerful antioxidant and anti-inflammatory herb that acts at multiple levels to generate these effects.[47,48]

Curcumin and its base molecules, called curcuminoids, are the subject of intense research at several major pharmaceutical companies that hope to capitalize on its apparently novel mechanisms. In addition to anti-inflammatory and antioxidant capacities, curcumin possesses characteristics more specific to AD. It appears to bind copper and iron to prevent the oxidative and beta-amyloid-producing effects of these metals.[49,50] Curcumin also appears to interfere with the formation of amyloid plaques once beta amyloid has been created as well as assist in the degradation of already-present plaques, thus acting on both sides of the beta-amyloid production and clearance equation.[51] Studies in animal models of AD have confirmed the therapeutic potential of curcumin. A number of studies have shown a decrease in beta-amyloid plaque formation and a decline in cognitive deficits in mice bred to develop AD.[52,53] One interesting study done on macrophages (immune cells) of human AD patients showed that these cells were ineffective at clearing beta-amyloid plaque, compared with controls, but when treated with curcumin, these cells cleared the plaque more effectively.[54] This effect of curcumin is additive to the similar effects generated by vitamin D. That is, combining curcumin with vitamin D produces effects greater than those produced by either supplement alone.[55]

In summary, curcumin is a powerful antioxidant and anti-inflammatory. It prevents oxidation by binding copper and iron, interferes with the formation of amyloid plaque and assists in clearing amyloid plaque from the brain. *Curcumin acts on at least four of our nine avenues.*

Ferulic Acid

Ferulic acid reduces oxidation and triggers production of protective proteins that fight brain-cell damage. Some of our nutritional elements in combating AD are in the class of polyphenols, compounds that wield antioxidant and anti-inflammatory effects, often exhibit anticancer benefits, and have specific additional effects in directly combating beta amyloid, cleavage of tau, and brain-cell death in general. Ferulic acid is structurally similar to polyphenols, but instead of containing two or more of the all-important structural component called the phenyl ring, its molecule contains only one. Nonetheless, it shares many beneficial nutritional attributes with polyphenols.

One of the anti-inflammatory effects of ferulic acid is to inhibit inflammatory protein 2, a mediator of inflammation that comes from white blood cells exposed to a well-studied, extremely inflammatory protein called TNF alpha.[56] In another test, brain cells in a tissue culture were exposed to beta amyloid, which induced a substantial increase in oxidative stress, including elevated protein and lipid oxidation followed by accelerated brain-cell death. Pretreatment of the brain cells with ferulic acid reduced the oxidation and stimulated genes that produced two key protective proteins: hemoxygenase-1 and heat shock protein 72. These proteins substantially minimized the brain-cell damage caused by the beta amyloid.[57] Several additional studies have corroborated these properties of ferulic acid and its ability to preserve brain cells under attack by beta amyloid both in vitro (test tube) and in laboratory animals.[58–61] *Ferulic acid, a phenolic nutritional supplement, affects at least three of our nine avenues.*

Ginger

The root and rhizome of the plant *Zingiber officinale* is commonly known as ginger. This herb has a number of medicinal applications and has been used as a medical treatment since ancient times. Ginger is well known for its anti-inflammatory and antinausea effects, but it also appears to possess complex properties that reach far into human physiology. Ginger may work against tumor cells, free radicals, and cell death as well as improve immune function.[62]

Ginger's effects on inflammation appear to involve numerous mechanisms.[63] Several studies have demonstrated that these complex mechanisms are indeed effective in fighting the inflammation provoked by beta-amyloid plaque and NFTs and in protecting brain cells from subsequent destruction.[64,65]

Additionally, ginger inhibits one of the enzymes that degrade the neurotransmitter acetylcholine (ACh) and may contribute to improved cognitive function through this mechanism as well.[66] This last mechanism is the same used by three of the FDA-approved medications for Alzheimer's disease. Blocking the degradation of ACh does boost the brain levels of this neurotransmitter, important for memory, but this benefit by itself is only temporary. *Our* reason for using ginger is its anti-inflammatory effect in *protecting* brain cells. *Ginger works along three of our nine avenues.*

American Ginseng

American ginseng, or *Panax quinquefolius*, is a well-known "adaptogen" herb, meaning it helps the body adapt to stress and balance or "tone" the various systems in the body. This herb has shown efficacy in preventing and treating upper-respiratory-tract infections and improving blood-glucose levels in diabetics.[67,68] It has also been reported to improve memory by increasing the activity of acetylcholine in the brain.[69,70] Since ancient times, various species of the genus *Panax* have been used to treat memory impairment. It may not be surprising, then, that several components (ginsenosides) of American ginseng appear to exert effects against the pathological processes of AD. Studies have shown that cells exposed to beta amyloid demonstrate signs of dysfunction and toxicity, hyper-phosphorylate tau protein to form NFTs, and may self-destruct (apoptosis), but that the application of American ginseng extract protected the cells from these effects.[71-76] Additionally, oral ginseng reduced beta-amyloid levels in the brains of test animals.[77]

Further still, ginseng compounds appear to reduce the cell dysfunction and toxicity that result from overexcitation by glutamate.[78] This is the intention of the prescription drug memantine (Namenda). Another study identified yet another mechanism showing that components of American ginseng significantly enhanced microglia-dependent scavenging of already-present beta amyloid.[79] In mouse models of "age-related" memory impairment, ginseng reduced memory impairment and beta-amyloid accumulation in the hippocampus and increased new brain-cell growth and rewiring (plasticity).[80,81] Thus, the data on American ginseng suggest that the root can fight formation of beta amyloid and NFTs, protect cells from the toxic effects of these abnormal proteins, prevent brain-cell death, protect brain cells from glutamate toxicity, help stimulate microglia to remove existing beta-amyloid plaque, and stimulate the generation of new brain cells and brain-cell connections. *American ginseng covers at least four of our nine avenues.*

Glycerylphosphorylcholine (GPC, Also Called Choline Alfoscerate)

A number of types of brain cells are affected in AD. These different cell types produce different neurotransmitters. (Neurotransmitters are the brain's communicators. They give the commands for our lungs to breathe, our hearts to beat, and our stomachs to digest our food.)

For people with AD, the cell type that makes the neurotransmitter called acetylcholine (ACh) is dysfunctional or missing. That's why early researchers focused on how to *increase* the secretion of ACh in the brains of AD patients. Most conventional drugs for AD are used because they increase ACh levels: These drugs work by inhibiting the enzymatic breakdown of ACh.

GPC can also increase ACh. Research on this supplement was intense before the widespread availability of AD pharmaceuticals, and by 2001 there had been at least thirteen published clinical trials examining 4,054 patients that cumulatively suggested that *GPC can significantly benefit dementia patients.*[82] More recently, a double-blind placebo-controlled trial of 400 mg of GPC each day in AD patients showed that those receiving the supplement continued to significantly improve in cognitive function over 180 days while the placebo group continued to decline in cognitive function over that time period.[83]

In summary, GPC proves beneficial by increasing levels of ACh but does not function specifically along any of our nine avenues. Nonetheless, we recommend it for its ACh effect because it is a natural nutrient with no side effects.

Green Tea/EGCG

You've no doubt heard by now that drinking green tea may benefit your health. Scientists have isolated many phytochemicals from the tea plant *Camellia senensis* (the source of green, white, black, and oolong teas). One of these chemicals is called epigallocatechin gallate (EGCG). It belongs to a larger class of chemicals called catechins, which are most abundant in green tea. EGCG has been marketed for a wide variety of purposes, including weight loss and cancer prevention. While that might seem far-reaching, research has confirmed that its usefulness may truly be this broad.

EGCG is known to have potent anti-inflammatory and anti-oxidative effects throughout the body, including within the brain, and these effects are mediated through multiple mechanisms on multiple levels.[84,85] EGCG and catechins also appear to bind iron and copper and reduce the pro-oxidative effects of these AD-associated metals.[86] Even more specific to AD, however, is EGCG's apparent ability to both increase alpha-secretase activity and decrease beta-secretase activity, leading to the production of benign soluble amyloid rather than the harmful beta amyloid.[87,88]

EGCG also seems to chip away at plaque from beta amyloid protein that has already been produced.[89] These impressive effects on the multifaceted pathways of AD have translated to protection against cognitive impairment in animal models of AD pathology or stroke.[90,91] *Green tea and green tea extract employ four of our nine avenues of attack.*

Medium Chain Triglycerides (MCTs)

MCTs, one type of saturated fat in coconut oil, appear to be useful in improving cognitive function in the case of Alzheimer's disease. In fact, a prescription version, called Axona, is now available and FDA-approved, but these fats are widely available in nature and in supplements that don't require a prescription. The benefit of MCTs for AD patients appears to be the ability of these fats to produce elevations of ketone bodies in the blood and brain; ketone bodies act as an alternative to glucose for fueling brain cells. Brain imaging and basic science studies reveal that glucose metabolism is impaired in AD patients, prompting some researchers to refer to AD as "type III diabetes." Ketone bodies, so the hypothesis goes, can increase brain-cell function by providing a more effective fuel.[92] Twenty grams of MCTs given daily to patients with either AD or mild cognitive impairment resulted in improved cognitive performance in patients who did not have the APOE4 genotype. To understand more about the APOE4 genotype, refer to the science text box below.

Alzheimer's and Genetics

There is a genetically transmitted form of AD that is rare compared with the common age-related and nearly epidemic AD. Those afflicted with the genetic form of AD are typically much younger at disease onset, often as young as forty.

For the common age-related AD, however, there is a genetic situation that does influence the risk of acquiring AD, the speed of progression, and the response to treatment. This is the configuration of a gene called APOE, a gene we all have. The gene has four components called alleles, named APO E1, E2, E3 and E4. APO E1 and E3 play no role in AD risk, but, simplistically speaking, APO E2 reduces risk and APO E4 increases both the risk and severity of AD.

We all have 2 copies of the APO E4 gene. If both copies contain E2, our risk is the lowest among the population. If we have one copy of E2 we have slightly reduced risk. If we have one copy of E4, we have increased risk and if we have two copies of E4 our risk is highest among our population and we'll be less responsive to treatment. When we refer to the APOE4 genotype, we're pinpointing individuals who have at least one copy of the E4 allele.

For unknown reasons, the benefit was very limited in those with the APOE4 genotype.[93] A larger study confirmed these results, again showing a significant improvement in cognitive function in APOE4-negative patients but not APOE4-positive patients. Further, the improvement was related to the level of beta hydroxybutyrate, a ketone body, and the improvement reversed upon discontinuation of the MCT product.[94] A study conducted in canine and murine (mouse) models of AD suggested that the benefits seen with MCTs (or a ketogenic diet that elevates ketone bodies) are mediated by an improvement in mitochondrial function (perhaps due to reduced oxidation or improved energy supply or both), as well as a reduction in APP and beta-amyloid production.[93,95] However, studies using ketogenic diets in a number of neurological disorders other than AD (such as Parkinson's disease, Lou Gehrig's disease (ALS), stroke, epilepsy, and traumatic brain injury) indicate that ketone bodies and beta-hydroxybutyrate specifically may provide more general neuroprotection. It is possible that the enhanced energy supply to brain cells allows the cells to more effectively deal with stresses and toxins and avoid cell death.[96]

The challenge of using MCTs for ketone production and, therefore, cognitive improvement is the possibility of gastrointestinal upset. This may occur in the form of bloating, cramping, or loose stool. To prevent this, simply start with a lower dose and build up gradually to develop tolerance to the gastrointestinal effect. Most people will need to start with 10 grams of MCTs taken once daily and work up to 20 grams as tolerated. If you notice bloating, cramping, or loose stool, reduce the dose and try increasing at a slower rate.

MCT oil can be purchased at most health-food stores or online. Additionally, coconut oil (100 percent pure or extra virgin) can be used to generate ketone bodies. To achieve 20 grams of MCTs from coconut oil, a dose of about 35 grams (35 ml) is needed.

We credit Mary Newport, MD, for recognizing the possible benefit of combining MCT oil and coconut oil. She has been using this combination to treat her husband's AD with apparent success. Her husband's blood results suggest that the peak ketone production from coconut oil may occur later than that of MCT oil, and the combination therefore may provide more sustained blood-ketone levels. Dr. Newport currently reports that her husband is receiving a whopping dose of 45 grams (45 ml) of a 1:1 ratio of MCT and coconut oil (22.5 grams each) three times a day, but his tolerance has been developed over nearly three years. *MCTs act along three of our nine avenues.*

Milk Thistle/Silymarin

This supplement has long been used to protect the liver from injury by chemicals and viruses. One likely mechanism is that it helps the liver (and body) to replenish glutathione, a major antioxidant in the body. Since oxidative stress and glutathione depletion have been implicated in several neurodegenerative diseases such as Alzheimer's disease and Parkinson's disease, it's not surprising that recent studies have shown that this supplement is effective in reducing the pathology of Alzheimer's disease. At least three studies have now shown that silymarin (or a component of silymarin called silibinin) can slow the production of beta amyloid and improve cognitive function in mouse models of Alzheimer's disease. The mechanisms appear to be the reduction in nitrogen free radicals (oxidative stress) and inflammation as well as the regeneration of glutathione in critical areas of the brain.[97–99] *Silymarin covers at least three of our nine avenues.*

N-Acetyl Cysteine (NAC)

This supplement has been the subject of research in a number of disciplines and for a number of conditions. The reason for such widespread interest is that NAC, like silymarin, helps to regenerate glutathione, one of the body's most abundant and powerful natural antioxidants. Since oxidative stress is involved in the development of AD, it is not surprising that this supplement has shown significant benefits in treating or preventing the disease. Cells from AD patients show abnormal levels of oxidation and a tendency to self-destruct, but NAC has proved able to minimize these abnormalities. The effect is more pronounced when combined with another molecule, alpha lipoic acid (discussed above).[100]

In patients with probable AD, NAC alone demonstrated impressive improvements in cognitive performance as measured by five different cognitive tests.[101] Further, NAC combined with B vitamins, vitamin E, acetyl-l-carnitine, and s-adenosyl-methionine led to twelve months of improving function in AD patients, followed by sixteen months of stable cognitive function.[102] The effects of NAC are not limited to glutathione regeneration. NAC helps to lower homocysteine levels (also lowered by B vitamins), which, as mentioned earlier in this chapter, is a risk factor for dementia, stroke, and heart disease and appears to contribute to formation of beta amyloid and NFTs.[103] *NAC functions along at least one and up to four of our avenues.*

Omega-3 Fatty Acids

Omega-3 fatty acids, and those from fish (DHA and EPA specifically), are now recognized to be critical for moderating inflammation in the body and for the normal function and development of cell membranes and tissues. The scientific evidence demonstrates that increasing omega-3 fatty acids from diet or supplements or both reduces the risk of heart disease, improves mood, eases inflammation, improves hormonal function, and reduces the risk of some cancers.[104] With such broad effects, then, it is no surprise that emerging evidence suggests a beneficial effect in preventing dementia and improving cognitive function. For example, one study demonstrated a 60 percent reduction in the diagnosis of Alzheimer's disease in patients eating at least one fish meal per week. The risk reduction was associated with the total intake of DHA, one of the major omega-3 fatty acids found in fish.[105]

This was reinforced in a 2010 review article that reported that people with a low level of DHA in the body were at an elevated risk for experiencing cognitive decline and developing AD.[106] Biochemical studies on DHA indicate that it does indeed exert effects on several of the fundamental processes of AD. DHA appears to inhibit oxidation, inflammation, and the phosphorylation of tau protein. It also improves insulin function and increases levels of brain-derived neurotrophic factor (BDNF). BDNF is a brain-protective protein that helps defend brain cells against the toxicity of beta amyloid and can also help grow new brain cells.[107] *Directly or indirectly, fish oil offers assistance on five of our nine avenues.*

Phosphatidylserine (PS)

The membranes of cells are made of fat molecules called phospholipids. These molecules provide precursors to various chemical mediators and determine membrane fluidity, which, in turn, affects the function of a number of hormones and other messengers. Phosphatidylserine is one such phospholipid and happens to be the most abundant phospholipid found in brain cells. Further, PS is a significant component of mitochondrial membranes, and mitochondrial dysfunction has been implicated in AD. PS has been the subject of at least twenty-three studies, twelve of which were double-blinded. The findings indicate that PS improves short-term memory, mood, concentration, and activities of daily living in patients with various forms of memory loss, including AD.[108–114] In addition to improving cell signaling and mitochondrial function, possible mechanisms include an increase in neurotransmitter secretion and production, the preservation of brain-cell connectivity (synaptogenesis), and the prevention of cell death (apoptosis).[108,115] *PS appears to be active on at least two of our nine avenues.*

Quercitin, Rutin, and Citrus Bioflavonoids

Bioflavonoids are a class of compounds prevalent in the leaves and skin of numerous fruits and vegetables. Quercitin and rutin are two closely related bioflavonoids. Bioflavonoids, particularly quercitin, demonstrate a plethora of favorable biological effects and help mediate many of the health benefits associated with fruit and vegetable consumption. Research has shown that quercitin or mixed bioflavonoids can fight inflammation and oxidation, prevent cancer-cell development, protect the heart and blood vessels, reduce histamine release (potentially helping to control allergies), inhibit viral infections, improve immune function, and alter metal metabolism.[116–119] There are plenty of reasons, therefore, to suspect that these compounds can influence the disease processes involved in AD. Research in this area has indeed shown activity more specific to AD. Remarkably, quercitin was able to stimulate growth of hippocampal neurons (cells from a brain area severely affected by AD) and restore losses in brain-cell connectivity that had been induced by beta amyloid.[120] Additionally, pretreatment of brain cells with quercitin protected these cells from the inflammation, oxidation, and self-destruction caused by beta-amyloid exposure.[121] Finally, quercitin, rutin, and related bioflavonoids have shown an interesting ability to prevent the accumulation of plaque from beta-amyloid protein by enhancing cell membrane characteristics.[122] *These remarkable nutritional compounds provide benefits along five of our nine avenues.*

Resveratrol (RSV)

The lower rate of cardiovascular disease among the French despite their higher rates of smoking and consumption of saturated fat is often referred to as the "French paradox." Because of the high rate of consumption of red wine in France, researchers began to analyze the many compounds found in red wine to explain this paradox. One of the compounds discovered is resveratrol (RSV). During times of stress, many plants, including grapes, produce protective molecules called phytoalexins, and RSV is one such protective molecule. Subsequent research on the molecule has shown that supplementation can replicate the beneficial effects of caloric restriction and increase longevity in animal models. In addition to enjoying enhanced longevity, these experimental animals demonstrated declines in cancers, inflammation, oxidation, insulin resistance, obesity, and cardiovascular disease.[123–126]

Mechanistic studies on RSV indicate that it may increase mitochondrial biogenesis (proliferation). Remember that mitochondria are the energy factories within cells, so increasing their ranks stands to improve energy availability to cells, helping them to withstand insults and remain healthy when challenged. This combination of effects (increased mitochondria along with reduced inflammation, oxidation, and insulin resistance) would suggest that RSV may be beneficial for the prevention and treatment of AD. Research specifically addressing the association between RSV and beta-amyloid plaque formation has, indeed, shown a reduction in plaque number as well as reductions in brain-cell oxidation and inflammation.[127–129]

The mechanisms behind these effects are complex and involve changes in gene expression.[130] In animal models, RSV has shown the ability to prevent cognitive decline and brain atrophy from both aging and toxin exposure.[131,132] In general, dosing was much higher than that provided by common supplement forms, and doses of approximately 1,400 mg daily for the average person may be needed if these effects are to fully translate to human subjects. This should be supplied specifically as *trans-resveratrol*; be careful of variances in terminology that can be deceptive. *At therapeutic doses, RSV has the potential to affect five of our nine avenues.*

Vitamin E, Vitamin C, and Beta-Carotene

These common micronutrients are often included in daily multivitamin supplements and maintain a favorable reputation among the public for their purported health benefits. While they play a critical role in numerous biochemical processes, debate continues as to whether these nutrients need to be supplemented or if adequate quantities can be obtained from a healthy diet alone. Many people take supplements of these nutrients simply because they doubt that their diet consistently provides optimal quantities of them. The antioxidant properties of these nutrients have resulted in their being examined for a relationship to degenerative diseases such as AD.

Several epidemiologic studies have confirmed an association between AD and low blood or tissue levels of vitamin E, vitamin C, and/or beta carotene.[133–136] Further, several well-done epidemiologic studies have indicated that elderly people who take supplements or have high dietary intake of these nutrients have a lower incidence of AD, while others have found no association.[137–141] Some epidemiologic studies have suggested that these associations may be explained simply by a reduced dietary intake of these nutrients (and most other nutrients) by AD patients.[142,143] However, more experimental studies have suggested that these nutrients may have a more direct effect on the root causes of cognitive impairment and AD.

Vitamin C (as ascorbic acid) has been shown to acutely improve cognitive function in mice and protect cells from oxidative insults.[144,145]

Vitamin E (as alpha-tocopherol) supplementation has been shown to significantly slow progression of cognitive decline in AD patients compared with controls, and with greater efficacy than the prescription antioxidant selegiline.[146] A study performed in mice demonstrated that vitamin E can reduce lipid oxidation and the deposition of amyloid plaque.[147] Gene-expression studies have shown that vitamin E is involved in regulating 948 genes, including those necessary for growth hormone, insulin-like growth factor I, brain-derived neurotrophic factor (BDNF), melatonin, dopamine, advanced glycation end product clearance, and beta-amyloid clearance.[148] All these activities would benefit the Alzheimer's brain. One study has implicated a negative effect of high-dose vitamin E (400 IU or more daily), specifically an increased rate of all-cause mortality.[149] This study has been criticized, however, because the form of vitamin E studied was d-alpha tocopherol only. In nature, in addition to alpha tocopherol, vitamin E from plants comes in the form of *mixed tocopherols*, including beta, gamma, and delta tocopherol as well as in a form called tocotrienols.

The daily dose of vitamin E (mixed and alpha-tocopherol) supplied by our Epigenetic Symphony powder is 280 IU. Not only does this supplement stay beneath the 400 IU dose that was implicated in increasing the all-cause mortality rate, but it is supplied as roughly equal amounts of d-alpha tocopherol and mixed tocopherols, providing what we believe is the perfect blend of effectiveness and safety.

Combining the above evidence would suggest that AD patients at the least have deficient intakes of these vital nutrients, and that supplementation can help compensate for this deficiency. Further, there is the possibility that supplementation will help slow the progression of cognitive impairment in AD patients in addition to providing adequate daily intakes. And available evidence would indicate that supplementation of vitamin E must be done with prudence and limited to doses below 400 IU daily.

Finally, smokers should not supplement beta-carotene, as studies have demonstrated a higher risk of lung cancer among this group. *This trio of antioxidants may function along four of our nine avenues.*

Medications with Root-Cause Effects

As we've discussed, for the most part the FDA-approved medications for Alzheimer's disease merely increase the production of the neurotransmitter acetylcholine in the brain for a temporary improvement in cognition while the underlying disease progresses. The only exception to this statement is the drug memantine (Namenda), which works by blocking a receptor in the brain called the

NMDA receptor. This interrupts the stimulation of these receptors by the molecule glutamate, effectively allowing the brain cells a bit of rest, which has resulted in temporary benefit. The purpose of this section is to discuss the benefit of two medications, not FDA-approved for AD, that appear to be very promising because they may influence the root causes of the disease.

Simvastatin

Simvastatin is a medication that is FDA-approved for cholesterol management. It is an inhibitor of the rate-limiting enzyme that manufactures cholesterol, called HMG CoA reductase. Like other medications in this class, called statins, it has a profound effect on cholesterol levels in the blood and has been shown to reduce heart-attack risk.

It has long been theorized, though, that statins work not just by improving one's cholesterol profile but also by providing a potent anti-inflammatory effect.[61] There are a good number of studies to substantiate this. We've referred to only one recent review article for the sake of simplicity because this is not a controversial issue and the review article, by Dr. Quist-Paulsen of the Norwegian University of Science and Technology, lists multiple original studies to support this concept. Population studies on the statins *as a medication class* are not convincing as to a beneficial effect on AD. However, most statin medications do not reach the brain because they are not fat-soluble and therefore cannot cross a membrane that extends from blood to brain called the blood-brain barrier.

As of this writing, only two statins have the ability to cross the blood-brain barrier into the brain: lovastatin and simvastatin. Lovastatin appears to be too weak in its effect to have anti-AD activity. Simvastatin, however, is much more potent. While the exact mechanism is unclear, simvastatin was demonstrated to be the only statin preventive for AD in a very large study (4.5 million participants). In this study, *simvastatin use was associated with a 50 percent reduction in the risk of developing AD.*[150] This finding held up even when the data were controlled for other confounding diseases that could be related to AD risk such as high blood pressure, heart disease, and diabetes. Whether the benefit comes from an anti-inflammatory effect in the brain is yet to be determined. Measurements of AD-related molecules in the cerebrospinal fluid after simvastatin treatment, however, suggest that this drug may at least inhibit the phosphorylation of tau protein, the necessary step in forming NFTs.[151] This benefit in prevention appears profound but does not necessarily translate into improvement for those already afflicted with AD. On the other hand, we believe it is probably of benefit when used with all our other elements. That said, the use of simvastatin is not for everyone, and the decision to use it should be individualized for each patient. Careful monitoring for side effects (muscle ache and liver irritation) is important here, requiring close supervision by a doctor.

Angiotensin-Converting Enzyme Inhibitors (ACEIs) and Angiotensin Receptor Blockers (ARBs)

ACEIs and ARBs are frequently used in the treatment of high blood pressure. Both types of drugs act on the renin-angiotensin-aldosterone system. This system is clearly involved in the regulation of blood pressure, but research suggests that its influence is much more broad.

In regard to AD, it is important to realize that, similar to statins, some of the specific ACEI drugs do not cross the blood-brain barrier while other drugs in this class do. Those specific ACEI drugs that do cross the blood-brain barrier and thus exert direct activity on the brain include captopril (Capoten), fosinopril (Monopril), lisinopril (Prinivil or Zestril), perindopril (Aceon), ramipril (Altace), and trandolapril (Mavik). These drugs are considered *centrally active* ACEIs.

In a study of 1,054 people, researchers found that for every year that a person was taking a centrally active ACEI, the rate of cognitive decline was reduced by 65 percent. In contrast, the incidence of dementia was increased 20 percent in those taking non–centrally active ACEIs.[152] Other studies have achieved similar findings, showing a dramatic reduction in cognitive decline from centrally active ACEI but no benefit from non–centrally active ACEI, other blood pressure medications, or no medication.[153,154]

Studies using animal models may give us an idea of how centrally active ACEIs support cognitive function. One study revealed that these drugs improved cognitive function in rats by improving cell density and capillary density (blood flow) in the hippocampus (the brain area involved in memory).[155]

Unlike some ACEIs, all ARBs are centrally active. Promising studies on ARBs and dementia suggest that they may be slightly more beneficial than ACEIs. A 2010 study published in the *British Medical Journal* demonstrated that those people taking ARBs had a 19 percent lower rate of AD than those taking the centrally active ACEI lisinopril and a 24 percent lower rate of AD than those taking other blood pressure medications.[156] Further, the benefits of the ARBs and lisinopril were additive, meaning that combining these drugs may offer protection beyond that provided by either one alone.

One possible reason ARBs appear to be more beneficial than ACEIs is that ARBs only target one angiotensin receptor (AT1) while ACEIs reduce the activity at both types of receptors (AT1 and AT2). It appears that the AT2 receptor mediates beneficial effects such as brain cell regeneration, so preserving the function of AT2 may be important.

Therefore, for those suffering from high blood pressure and with a concern about cognitive impairment and dementia, we recommend asking your doctor for an ARB. Common ARBs include candesartan (Atacand), losartan (Cozaar), and telmisartan (Micardis). For those without high blood pressure but at risk of (or diagnosed with) dementia, discuss the use of a low-dose ARB with your physician, who will need to monitor your blood pressure to make sure it does not drop too low. In either case, it may be prudent to combine a low dose of an ARB with a low dose of a centrally active ACEI. This will become clearer in the near future as the evidence continues to accumulate.

Nonsteroidal Anti-Inflammatory Drugs (NSAIDs)

NSAIDs include common over-the-counter anti-inflammatory drugs like ibuprofen, naproxen, and aspirin as well as some prescription drugs like celecoxib (Celebrex) and meloxicam (Mobic). There is currently a great deal of research investigating the usefulness of this drug class in the prevention or treatment of AD, but the results are far from conclusive and are often contradictory. Some studies have shown that these drugs can actually increase the incidence of dementia or activate mechanisms thought to contribute to AD, though questions about methodology, bias, and confounding remain. *Due to the uncertainty surrounding these drugs' effect on the progression of AD and the potential adverse effects of this drug class, their use is not consistent with the Leonardi Institute's commitment to effective or possibly effective interventions with the highest degree of safety and minimal adverse effects.* However, the research examining NSAIDs and their effect on AD will be followed for new developments.

STEP 4: Summary of Recommendations

Take the following nutritional supplements that support brain function and/or specifically combat the root causes of AD. Ideally, our recommended daily dose should be taken as half that amount, twice a day, with food.

Our patients appreciate the convenience of having items one to twenty-four in our powdered drink mix, Epigenetic Symphony, which substantially simplifies taking most of these beneficial supplements. Items twenty-five through thirty-two were not included in the Epigenetic Symphony formula. In some cases this was due to the difficulty in producing a dry form, in others it was for taste considerations and in the case of phytate cream, due to the requirement of skin application as opposed to oral use. We therefore provide these items as separate supplements. We also offer a discounted supplement kit that includes everything on this list (except the prescription items - #33 below and the MCT oil - #31 below) through our nutritional supplement website, www.Cycle-breakers. com. The kit is called Illuminate!™. For prescription items, you will need to see your physician or one of our specialists in Denver. For the MCT oil, on our website we recommend another vendor only because they can provide a quality product at a lower price than we're able to.

But you can also assemble these ingredients on your own. Please be careful to distinguish between milligrams (mg) and micrograms (mcg)—1 mg equals 1,000 mcg.

1. Vitamin B6, 100 mg (milligrams)

2. Vitamin B12, 360 mcg (micrograms)

3. Vitamin C, 1,000 mg

4. Vitamin D, 5,000 IU (international units)

5. Vitamin E, 280 IU (from both mixed tocopherols and d-alpha tocopherol)

6. Acetyl-l-carnitine (ALCAR), 3,000 mg

7. Alpha-lipoic acid (ALA), 350 mg

8. Beta carotene, 10,000 IU (avoid this if you smoke)

9. Citrus bioflavonoids, 1,500 mg

10. Biotin, 3,000 mcg

11. Choline bitartrate, 200 mg

12. Chromium polynicotinate, 600 mcg

13. Folic acid, 2 mg

14. Garlic extract, 8 mg (from freeze-dried powder)

15. Ginger, 1,500 mg

16. Ginseng (American), 1,500 mg

17. Green tea extract, 1,500 mg

18. N-acetyl cysteine, 1,500 mg

19. Rutin, 600 mg

20. Selenium, 100 mcg

21. Quercitin, 200 mg

22. Ferulic acid, 100 mg

23. Milk thistle extract, 750 mg (standardized to 80% silymarin)

24. Vitamin B3 as nicotinamide, 1,400 mg

25. Caffeine, 300–500 mg per day, from coffee if it does not cause insomnia.

26. Curcumin, 1,400 mg, together with Bioperine, 70 mg for optimal absorption

27. Trans resveratrol, 1,400 mg

28. Glycerylphosphorylcholine, 1,000 mg

29. Phosphatidyl serine, 100 mg

30. Fish oil containing 1,200 mg EPA and 800 mg DHA

31. Medium chain triglycerides (MCTs) or MCT/coconut oil mix: 20 grams MCTs all at once, one to three times daily

32. Fifty percent phytate cream or gel for skin application, ¼ tsp daily rubbed into skin

33. Simvastatin, ARB, and ACEI as medically appropriate.

STEP 5   The Importance of Hormones for Your Brain

Safely Maintaining Healthy Hormone Levels

I s it a coincidence that hormone levels *decline* with age while Alzheimer's disease *increases* with age?

When two events occur at the same time, it doesn't prove that one causes the other. But the association between hormone levels and Alzheimer's disease is strong enough to prompt curious scientists to investigate the possibility of cause and effect. We reviewed all the available scientific evidence about the relationship among aging, AD, and hormones so that we could help our patients avoid and combat the negative effects of hormone depletion.

Hormones are chemical messengers that are made and released by glands called endocrine glands. Hormones have powerful effects on many organs in our bodies, including our brains. Anyone who's raised a teenager can attest to this!

Examples of hormones include cortisol, thyroid hormone, insulin, melatonin, the male hormones testosterone and DHEA, and the female hormones estradiol and progesterone. Vitamin D is also technically a hormone.

As we discuss the hormones throughout this chapter, it's important to keep in mind that male hormones are not unique to men, nor are female hormones unique to women. Male hormones have important functions in women, and female hormones have important functions in men.

How Hormones Affect Alzheimer's Disease

As our bodies age from oxidative stress, glycation, inflammation, sleep deprivation, chronic stress, and lifestyle errors, our endocrine glands age, too. The result is a gradual decline in a number of vital hormones. Believe it or not, this decline begins as early as age thirty. For example, around that age, testosterone levels begin to decline by an average of about 1 percent a year. DHEA declines twice as fast—by about 2 percent a year. Melatonin drops by about 80 percent sometime between its peak at age thirteen and age thirty-five. Estradiol and progesterone undergo a very gradual decline in women throughout adult life but most noticeably at menopause, when levels drop to nearly zero over several years. This is important information because hormones influence the function of our brain cells and their overall health.

Let's take a look at the hormones that most influence Alzheimer's disease and how that influence occurs.

Testosterone

Testosterone is an important male hormone responsible for male sexual development, secondary sex characteristics, lean mass, bone density, sex drive, sexual performance, and many other functions, including some in the brain. Based on the evidence we cite below, it is clear that the normal decline in testosterone that occurs with age is one of the many factors in the development of AD.

Testosterone Benefits in AD

▶ Reduces beta-amyloid production

▶ Enhances beta-amyloid breakdown and removal

▶ Protects brain cells from the beta amyloid already present

▶ Reduces the cleavage of tau to prevent neurofibrillary tangles

The Science of Testosterone in AD

In population studies of normal men, those with higher testosterone levels were shown to have better cognitive function than those with lower levels.[1,2] In clinical trials of testosterone replacement, normal aging men with testosterone levels at the lower end of the normal range experienced improvements in both verbal and spatial memory when the level was raised to the upper normal range.[3] Interestingly, there was no benefit if the testosterone level was raised either very slightly or too high (above normal). The sweet spot was *upper normal*. But how about men with Alzheimer's? Well, testosterone replacement was also very effective in improving both verbal and spatial memory in a study of men with either Alzheimer's or mild cognitive impairment (pre-Alzheimer's).[4]

Meanwhile, as our testosterone levels decline with age, the levels of another hormone called luteinizing hormone (LH) rise. LH's job is to stimulate more testosterone production. It makes sense that it rises as testosterone drops, because the body senses the reduced testosterone level and is trying to compensate by increasing testosterone production. It just so happens that as LH levels rise, levels of beta-amyloid protein in the blood also rise.[5] How do we reduce the level of LH to bring the blood levels of beta amyloid down? We supplement testosterone!

That reduces *blood* levels of beta amyloid, but how about reducing *brain* levels? Well, testosterone influences brain levels of beta amyloid through two other hormones: dihydrotestosterone (DHT) and estradiol (a female hormone). Some of the testosterone in both men and women is converted by the body into these other two hormones. So the more testosterone we have, the more DHT and estradiol our bodies can make. Both DHT and estradiol influence brain beta amyloid by stimulating the activity of an enzyme called neprilysin.[6,7] Neprilysin cleaves beta amyloid into smaller, more soluble components that can be removed from the brain. Estradiol also eliminates beta amyloid by multiple mechanisms that we'll discuss in the estradiol section below.

Beta amyloid (the harmful protein) comes from the cleavage of amyloid precursor protein (APP) by the enzyme *beta* secretase. When APP is cleaved by an enzyme called *alpha* secretase, a harmless soluble form of amyloid—*alpha* amyloid—is made. Testosterone has been shown to increase the production of alpha amyloid at the expense of production of beta amyloid.[8] To put it simply, testosterone reduces the production of beta amyloid in the brain.

Ready for another one? We've already discussed how the cleavage of tau protein leads to neurofibrillary tangles. One important enzyme that cleaves tau protein is called calpain. Testosterone also blocks calpain, inhibiting NFT formation.[9] In an extension of this finding, the reduction in NFT formation by testosterone was further confirmed to improve brain-cell survival.[9]

Finally, testosterone has been shown to protect brain cells from the toxicity of beta amyloid by increasing the production of a brain-protective protein called HS Protein 70.[10]

That's just one hormone that addresses four of our nine avenues. Furthermore, it's been proved that low testosterone is a risk factor for cognitive decline and that testosterone replacement improves cognitive function in both normal people and AD patients. One might begin to think that testosterone alone might be able to reverse AD, but remember, it's only one of the thirty elements we're recommending.

Estradiol

Estradiol is the most potent human estrogen. It's produced in the ovary, so at menopause, when the ovaries get their gold watch, estradiol levels plummet to near zero. Many problems and symptoms occur around menopause that are outside the scope of this book. Here we'll focus only on AD-related issues, which are many.

Estradiol has been shown to combat Alzheimer's disease by even more avenues than testosterone.

Estradiol Benefits in AD

▶ Estradiol, in addition to testosterone, increases the production of alpha amyloid, reducing beta-amyloid production.[11]

▶ Estradiol, in addition to DHT, enhances activity of the enzyme neprilysin, helping to break down and remove beta amyloid from the brain.[7]

▶ Estradiol increases the activity of two other enzymes that break down beta amyloid. These are insulin-degrading enzyme (IDE)[12] and transthyretin.[13]

▶ Like testosterone, estradiol boosts the production of HSP 70, protecting brain cells from the beta amyloid already present in the brain.[10]

Here are more findings to support the benefit of estradiol for Alzheimer's disease.

▶ Postmenopausal women with AD had lower levels of estradiol in their spinal fluid than women without AD.[14]

▶ Cognitive test scores of women with estradiol levels in the lowest 33 percent declined faster than those in the highest 33 percent.[15]

▶ Women with AD who were treated with estradiol gel applied to the skin improved relative to those given a placebo.[16]

▶ In one study of men, testosterone replacement improved both spatial and verbal memory, but verbal memory improved only in men whose estradiol level rose 80 percent in response to the higher testosterone level (a common event since, in men, estradiol is made from testosterone).[17] Here's one area where the physician's experience and expertise is extremely important. When a topical testosterone skin cream is given to men, the estradiol level rises along with the testosterone level (typically about 80 percent). This is good for the brain but is not high enough to cause feminine characteristics such as breast growth. However, if the testosterone is injected, estradiol levels typically rise to very high levels, often causing breast soreness or breast growth in men. This can be controlled with certain medications *if* the doctor is aware of the issue and skilled in its control. At the very least, blood levels of testosterone and estradiol must be monitored and the estradiol level controlled when needed.

While there is more evidence than we've presented here, we believe you have enough of a picture to be convinced of the substantial benefit of estradiol replacement for AD. But what about safety? For a thorough discussion regarding the safety of bioidentical hormone replacement after menopause, we refer you to the appendix at the end of the book.

Bioidentical Hormone Replacement Therapy (BHRT) along with the other aspects of our program is designed to help our Alzheimer's patients enjoy an improvement in intellect and either arrest or reverse their disease, potentially adding decades of high-quality life. This is our mission, and we are very determined.

When administered judiciously, with proper monitoring of blood levels along with regular screening, BHRT is both safe and extremely effective. And estradiol, being very protective against AD, is an important component of our overall program.

Progesterone

Progesterone is the most prominent female hormone after estradiol. Progesterone is considered the hormone of pregnancy. High levels occur during pregnancy, and without those high levels, pregnancies cannot be maintained. But is there a role for progesterone after menopause? The answer is a resounding yes.

Progesterone Benefits in AD

When properly administered in cyclical fashion, progesterone has the following important benefits:

▶ Works on at least three of our avenues of attack

▶ Augments the benefits of estradiol

▶ Appears to combat the depression that often accompanies AD

First, progesterone is a necessity in BHRT for women who haven't had hysterectomies, because it protects the uterus from endometrial cancer. For women on estrogen replacement along with progesterone, the risk of uterine cancer is no higher than for women not using HRT at all. In addition, progesterone is a very important bone-building hormone, protecting postmenopausal women from osteoporosis. For this reason, we at the Leonardi Institute use progesterone even for women who have had hysterectomies.

Now let's look at the evidence for the role of progesterone specifically for AD.

1. In a study of postmenopausal mice that were bred to develop Alzheimer's, estrogen slowed the production of beta-amyloid protein. When progesterone was administered continuously, it blocked this benefit. However, when progesterone was administered cyclically (on and off), the estrogen benefit was actually enhanced.[18]

2. In another study in mice bred to develop AD, progesterone curbed depression-related behavior.[19] Depression is often a serious component of Alzheimer's, and improvement provides great comfort to both patients and family.

3. The Department of Pharmacology and Neuroscience at the University of North Texas Health Science Center at Fort Worth conducted a study to compare bioidentical progesterone with the synthetic medroxyprogesterone. Only the bioidentical progesterone was shown to increase brain levels of BDNF, the important protein that stimulates development of new brain cells and helps establish connections between brain cells.[20]

4. In another study of mice bred to develop AD, progesterone was instrumental in slowing the phosphorylation of tau protein, the beginning of the process in the development of the neurofibrillary tangles.[21]

Since men normally have very low levels of progesterone, progesterone is not supplemented in men.

Melatonin

Melatonin is a hormone produced by the pineal gland during deep sleep. It is commonly known as the hormone that regulates circadian rhythm (day/night, sleep/awake cycle). But melatonin also acts as an antioxidant and a cancer inhibitor.

Melatonin Benefits in AD

▶ Works on at least four of our nine avenues of attack

▶ Can diminish oxidative damage

▶ Rescues brain cells from self-destruction (apoptosis)

New research demonstrates a link among sleep deficiency, cognitive impairment, and AD. The mechanisms behind these associations are multiple, but melatonin deficiency is probably one of them. Here are the findings of some studies relating melatonin to AD specifically:

1. Melatonin has been shown to prevent cell damage induced by beta amyloid in the hippocampus of the brain. The hippocampus is the primary memory region of the brain and the area most affected by AD. Melatonin also combats inflammation and the phosphorylation of tau protein.[22]

2. Mice bred to develop AD were fed aluminum to increase brain damage via oxidative stress. Mice that were also given melatonin exhibited greatly reduced oxidation in the brain in response to the aluminum.[23]

3. Melatonin can reduce oxidative damage within the mitochondria (energy factories) of brain cells and rescue the brain cells from self-destruction.[24] This self-destruction, or apoptosis, of brain cells is a common final pathway in a number of neurodegenerative diseases, including Alzheimer's disease, Parkinson's disease, Huntington's

disease, and amyotrophic lateral sclerosis (ALS, or Lou Gehrig's disease). Melatonin has been shown to slow cell destruction in all of these conditions.[25]

4. The brain cell-protective effects of melatonin are not just mediated through its antioxidant properties but also through its influence on gene products called sirtuins, which tend to improve the function and longevity of cells.[26]

5. Melatonin's protective effects on brain-cell mitochondria appear to be more pronounced in younger people, underscoring its effectiveness in prevention.[27] In terms of treatment, we consider it a critical component of our program.

Vitamin D3

Vitamin D is technically not a vitamin at all. Vitamin D3, or cholecalciferol, is technically a hormone and acts on hormone receptors within nearly all cells in the body. The term *vitamin* refers to an essential nutrient that we cannot manufacture in our bodies, but we can and do make vitamin D. It is synthesized through the action of several enzymes in the body as a result of skin exposure to ultraviolet radiation (sunlight). Additionally, humans obtain a portion of their necessary vitamin D through dietary intake. Vitamin D deficiency or insufficiency is extremely common throughout the world. Deficiency has been associated with an increased incidence of osteoporosis, rickets, cancer, autoimmune disease, viral infections, hypertension, insulin resistance, and fibromyalgia.[28] Therefore, correcting a vitamin D deficiency is important for health in general. Additionally, impressive evidence is accumulating that suggests vitamin D may be important for preventing and treating cognitive impairment and Alzheimer's disease as well.

Further, vitamin D stimulates macrophages, immune cells that are thought to play a role in the clearance of beta-amyloid plaque from the brain. Another of our recommended supplements, curcumin, was discussed in Step 4. Curcumin also stimulates macrophages to remove beta amyloid. Another important finding is that when vitamin D and curcumin are combined, the stimulatory effect on macrophages is greater than when either is used alone. That is to say, the two supplements are additive in benefit.[29]

Vitamin D Benefits in AD

▶ People with lower vitamin D intake are significantly more likely to have cognitive impairment.[30]

▶ Alzheimer's patients appear to have lower vitamin D levels than people without the disease.[31]

DHEA

DHEA is the abbreviation for the hormone dehydroepiandrosterone. Like estradiol, testosterone, and progesterone, DHEA is a steroid hormone. The media might lead you to believe that the term *steroid* refers to an illegal hormone used by overzealous athletes. In truth, *steroid* is a scientific term that refers to the chemical structure of a compound and basically means the compound is made in the body from cholesterol.

DHEA Benefits in AD

▶ Improves both the survival and growth of young brain cells

▶ May improve learning and memory

▶ Directly inhibits the activity of beta secretase, inhibiting beta-amyloid formation

DHEA is a male hormone, but like testosterone it is very prevalent in both men and women. It is made in the adrenal glands, which sit atop each kidney. When taken by mouth, DHEA is absorbed well into the bloodstream and is quickly sulfated (a sulfate group is attached) to form DHEA-sulfate, or DHEAS.

DHEAS levels are easily measured in a blood test, and these levels decline with age by more than 2 percent a year.

Let's look at the evidence behind the use of DHEA to prevent or treat AD:

1. Alzheimer's victims have lower levels of DHEAS than age-matched controls, and the volume of the hippocampus, the memory area of the brain most affected by AD, becomes smaller as DHEAS levels decline.[32]

2. As we discussed in Step 2, inflammation is one of the primary mechanisms that destroy brain cells. Chemicals that mediate this inflammation are called cytokines. One such cytokine is called interleukin 2 (IL2). IL2 stimulates immune cells called natural killer cells to attack brain cells, and this process is accelerated in AD. However, incubating AD patients' natural killer cells with DHEA tempered the cells' overactive response to IL2, rendering them potentially less harmful.[33]

3. A 2010 study of adult mice showed that beta-amyloid protein worked against the survival of new brain cells that were forming but that treatment with DHEA aided both the survival and growth of the young brain cells.[34]

4. One of the ways beta-amyloid protein kills brain cells is by opening calcium channels in the cell, flooding the cell with so much calcium that the cell dies. Investigators in Japan showed that pretreating the cells with DHEA decreased the calcium flux into the cells by the beta amyloid.[35]

5. DHEAS was able to improve learning and memory in mice bred to develop AD.[36]

6. A protein called VEGF promotes the development of new blood vessels in the brain as well as delivery of nutrients to brain cells. VEGF activity is impaired in AD patients compared with healthy people and even compared with patients with vascular dementia. When the cells that make VEGF were incubated in DHEA, VEGF production increased.[37]

7. In a study that confirmed the lower levels of DHEA in brains of AD patients, those lower levels also correlated with higher levels of hyperphosphorylated tau and beta-amyloid accumulation.[38] Furthermore, beta amyloid accumulated in the specific areas of the brain where DHEA activity was lowest.

8. We discussed earlier how oxidative stress promotes the cleavage of amyloid precursor protein by the enzyme beta secretase to form the toxic beta-amyloid protein in the brain. DHEA has been shown to directly inhibit the activity of beta secretase, inhibiting beta-amyloid formation.[39]

Human clinical trials aimed at improving cognition in older adults with DHEA, however, are not convincing. Of three studies in particular, one on postmenopausal women demonstrated improvement[40] while another resulted in cognitive decline[41] and yet another on both men and women showed no effect.[42] Keep in mind, though, that conflicting trials are common in medicine, and we've emphasized throughout this book that no single agent is a magic bullet. Again, this is the reason we're employing multiple agents to affect as many of our nine avenues as possible. For DHEA, we have evidence for activity along five of our nine avenues.

The Proper Dose of DHEA

The dose of DHEA is predicated on baseline blood level and should be adjusted by a physician based on follow-up levels. The dose ranges from 10 mg to 200 mg, depending on the blood level during treatment. For men, we recommend a level of 350 to 500 µg/dl, and for women, we recommend a level of 250 to 400 µg/dl (1 µg/dl = .001 mg/dl).

The most common side effect of DHEA is acne, and it's more common in women than in men. If you develop acne, stop the DHEA until the acne clears up. Once your skin is clear, you can resume the DHEA at about half your previous dose. If the acne recurs, continue to reduce the dose until you find the dose at which you can maintain clear skin.

STEP 5: Summary of Recommendations

▶ Undertake optimal hormone replacement under the care of a physician skilled in the art. Women should consider bioidentical estrogen, progesterone, DHEA, melatonin, vitamin D3, and testosterone. The estrogen should be administered only via the skin (never by mouth). Men should consider bioidentical DHEA, melatonin, vitamin D3, and testosterone.

▶ Blood levels of estradiol, testosterone, and DHEA-sulfate should be monitored in both men and women and doses adjusted accordingly. For women, progesterone should also be monitored, and for men, dihydrotestosterone (DHT) should also be monitored.

▶ For melatonin, blood levels need not be monitored. Since melatonin promotes deeper levels of sleep, we adjust the dose according to how well a patient is sleeping. A typical dose is 3 mg at bedtime, but it can be widely adjusted based on sleep. Remember, though, that the primary purpose of melatonin is not for sleep but for its benefit in four of our nine avenues involving the brain. Therefore, even if it's not needed to aid sleep, we still administer 3 mg at bedtime.

STEP 6   Improve Your Brain Power
Brain Aerobics, Meditation, & Sleep

While being diagnosed with AD can often make people feel like they're no longer in control of their lives, you now know from reading Steps 1 through 5 that there are a lot of actions you can take to prevent and reverse this disease. As we said in the introduction, all the steps are equally important, and Step 6 is no exception. The assignments we give you in this chapter are every bit as critical to your success as the other five steps.

Brain Aerobics

People who regularly engage in focused cognitive activity are at a lower risk of developing dementia of any type, including AD.[1-3] Equally important, increasing cognitive activity after a diagnosis of cognitive impairment or dementia can significantly slow progression of the disease.[4] So as the saying goes, it's time to put on your thinking cap!

Focused cognitive activity simply means focused thinking, learning, and problem-solving. If you are retired and not actively involved in a business, a workplace, or an intellectually challenging hobby, engaging in brain aerobics is even more essential. *Focused cognitive activities include the following*:

▶ Learning new information or skills

▶ Studying a foreign language

▶ Learning to play a musical instrument

▶ Working on crossword puzzles

▶ Solving math problems

▶ Deciphering riddles

▶ Playing board games or card games that require strategy

▶ Taking up a new hobby

The activities can be work-related, educational, or recreational. The key is to do something that truly involves focused attention and thinking on a regular basis, and preferably every day.

The opposite of focused cognitive activity is called *passive thought*. This would include planning your dinner while driving the car, daydreaming, watching television, and lying in bed awake with your mind jumping from one thought to another or worrying about your problems.

Cognitive activity can increase levels of brain-derived neurotrophic factor (BDNF), which protects brain cells from the toxicity of beta-amyloid protein and stimulates the growth of new brain cells.[5,6] Cognitive activity can also help rewire the brain circuitry and work around dysfunctional areas (a phenomenon known as neuroplasticity). This phenomenon is behind just about all types of learning.

In the case of AD, cognitive exercise or training can lead to improved cognitive function by maximizing the brain-cell connections involved in various mental tasks. These connections are like bridges—the more bridges, the less likely traffic will come to a standstill when one goes down. More brain cells and increased connectivity between those cells lead to what researchers call increased *cognitive reserve*. Cognitive reserve is like muscle strength—it can be increased through training.

Therefore, we have created a series of cognitive exercises we call *brain aerobics*. These exercises are intended to increase cognitive reserve. This list of exercises is meant to offer a start to cognitive reserve training, but because the exercises are to be practiced daily, this short list can get monotonous. It is recommended that each patient work with a caregiver, partner, or friend to expand on this list and create similar or related exercises that are both challenging and enjoyable. Creating new exercises is in itself a cognitive exercise.

Mental Exercises for Improving Cognitive Function

Practice one or more exercises each day, making sure to rotate through the list and cover all exercises with regularity. Several exercises may require interaction with or help from another person. These are not meant to be easy, so please don't get discouraged.

1. Reminisce about the past (three different exercises).
   a. Tell stories about favorite childhood activities or events.
   b. Recall all your childhood and young-adult friends, and relate stories as the memories emerge.
   c. Recall remarkable experiences in your life.

2. Account for the current circumstances (place of residence, occupation, marital status, number of children, etc.) of all your siblings, children, and extended relatives.

3. Name as many US presidents as possible. Give additional details regarding their presidencies if possible.

4. Name as many vegetables, fruits, cars, trees, or flowers as possible.

5. Have an assistant make up and tell a short story (three or four sentences), and then recite the story or recall as many details as possible. Then make up a short story of your own. Have your assistant recite the story to you and check your assistant for accuracy.

6. Pick a letter of the alphabet and name all the words you can think of (excluding proper names) that begin with that letter.

7. Talk about one of your favorite books.

8. Use your imagination to describe the most perfect or exciting paradise. Develop a fictional story around it. Make one of the characters possess great wisdom.

9. Using a standard deck of cards, separate the suits (spades, diamonds, clubs, and hearts) into four stacks.

10. Attempt to build a house of cards.

11. Find puzzles and games such as crossword puzzles and memory games, and work with a friend to complete them.

12. Have an assistant place the numbers 1–15 and the letters A–O randomly on an 8.5-by-11-inch sheet of paper, using the entire surface and avoiding any particular pattern. Your task is to connect the numbers and letters, in sequence, beginning with a number and alternating between letters and numbers. For example, start with 1, connect with a line to A, and then connect with a line to 2, then to B, and so on, until you end with O. Reverse positions and create the numbers and letters for your assistant to connect.

Mindfulness

Mindfulness is a type of meditation that can improve elements of cognition. It could be argued that practicing mindfulness is a cognitive exercise and could easily have been included above in the "brain aerobics" section. However, to Westerners, mindfulness is a unique and often-foreign way of experiencing the world, and therefore it deserves its own discussion. We strongly advise mindfulness or another variety of meditation for everyone.

Mindfulness is a state of mind or state of being in which observation or thought is conducted with patience, acceptance, and curiosity and *without* judgment. The term *beginner's mind* is often used to describe mindfulness, because the experience is very similar to observing a completely unfamiliar object or event. It's nearly impossible to judge and respond with negative emotion to something completely unfamiliar.

Imagine yourself looking at a small, strange, and nonthreatening object. Notice how a sense of curiosity, heightened awareness, and nonjudgmental observation dominate the experience. Also notice how this awareness is of the present moment or, in fact, of no moments whatsoever. You are experiencing the here and now, which is dynamic and always changing.

It could also be said that mindfulness is a preconceptual experience. Mindful awareness is naturally present before judgments and determinations are made; your goal is to draw out and dwell in this preconceptual experience. The experience is not of a tree, for example, but of the entity that we label a tree and *all* the circumstances that are manifesting the "present-moment" sensation of this entity. Thus, it's not the trunk, branches, bark, leaves, scents, sunlight, warmth, grass, wind, birds chirping, clouds, gravity, and breath that one experiences but the "bloom" (as Thoreau said) of one or more of these entities before these labels are given.

Mindfulness is not limited to our environment (external awareness) and can easily be focused on the body, on thoughts, or on pain or other sensations (internal awareness). The next time you injure yourself, mindfully experience the pain and notice the richness of this sensory experience. Notice how it is not negative or positive, just intriguing and phenomenal. The goal is to adopt this disposition toward the entire experience of life's events, people, thoughts, and sensations. It takes regular practice but becomes more automatic with time. The obvious result is limited stress and anxiety and a richer, more engaging experience of life.

Additionally, several studies on mindfulness practice have noted benefits directly related to cognitive function and brain-tissue density. Practicing mindfulness appears to significantly increase attentional capacity, visuo-spatial processing, working memory, and executive function, even after only four days of training.[7-10] These results suggest that the benefits may be mediated by pattern changes in brain-cell connectivity, coordination, and activity.

Long-term mindfulness meditators have been shown to have greater thickness in their brain's cortex (brain-cell area) than non-meditators have, suggesting the ability to produce changes in the brain's physical structure as well.[11] Possible mechanisms would include protecting brain cells from death (preventing atrophy), increasing the growth of new brain cells, increasing brain vasculature (the blood-flow network), and expanding brain-cell branching (arborization).

Another possible mechanism behind the improvements in cognitive function and cortical thickness that are seen with mindfulness might simply be a reduction of stress. Simply living in the hyperstimulating environment of US cities, watching the news media's paranoid reports, working to meet deadlines and stay on top of both work and personal commitments, and even physical activity without adequate rest and recovery can damage the body, including the brain.

Stress, whether it's physical, mental, or emotional, engages the sympathetic arm of our nervous system that causes us to fight, flee, or freeze. The other arm of our nervous system, called the parasympathetic arm, is responsible for digestion, rest, and recovery. When we are healthy, the parasympathetic arm keeps the sympathetic arm in check. Our health depends on the oscillating balance between these two arms of our physiology. Therefore, stress and anxiety are not innately bad or harmful when they are short-lived and balanced with rest, recovery, and good digestion. So, "balanced stress" is healthy and unbalanced stress is unhealthy.

Most Americans, however, experience chronic stress, and the sympathetic arms of their nervous systems are dominant. The sympathetic arm releases epinephrine (adrenaline), norepinephrine, and cortisol into the body. These neurotransmitters and hormones cause blood-vessel constriction, elevated blood pressure, elevated heart rate, shallow and rapid breathing, muscular tension, irritability, aggression, and anxiety. These consequences, in turn, are associated with nearly all degenerative diseases, including heart attacks, strokes, dementia, diabetes, and cancers. Sympathetic dominance is also a major contributor to chronic conditions like irritable bowel syndrome and gastric reflux disease, and it suppresses the immune system, leading to an increased vulnerability to infectious diseases.

The elevation in cortisol that occurs with chronic stress may be specifically related to dementia and AD. When elevated chronically or to very high levels, cortisol becomes toxic to brain cells. It especially damages the area of the brain associated with memory formation (the hippocampus) and the fear response (the amygdala). Damage to these areas is the suspected cause of post-traumatic stress disorder (PTSD) and also leads to atrophy (shrinkage) of the hippocampus. The result can be cognitive dysfunction and impairment.

Mindfulness is a powerful intervention for managing and mitigating stress. Much of what causes stress is not reality but a fabrication of possible realities by our minds. The immediate consequence is two-sided: We create worry, fear, anger, and judgment while simultaneously failing to experience *real* life. The long-term consequences are innumerable and include almost all degenerative diseases, including dementia. There are many good books on the subject, among them Jon Kabat-Zinn's books written for the Western public. His book *Wherever You Go, There You Are* is a good place to start.

Social Engagement and Activity

There is also evidence to suggest that social activity may be beneficial in regard to preventing or improving dementia.[12] The research is not clear on whether the benefit comes from cognitive activity (since social activity is often associated with planning, games, and reminiscing), physical activity (since socializing is often associated with walking, dancing, etc.), or actual social connections and relationships. It *is* well-known that social withdrawal and depression often accompany AD. That's one reason that AD patients and caregivers can benefit tremendously from support groups and connection to others who are experiencing the same challenges.

As part of our comprehensive treatment program, we recommend maintaining social activity as much as possible and seeking out local and national AD support groups and organizations. Social activity does not need to be limited to well-attended events. Simply having regular visits with a few caring family members and friends can be extremely beneficial.

Sleep

It is absolutely clear that sleep is critical for our health, including cognitive health and memory formation. Unfortunately, few people (including many doctors and scientists) seem to know how important sleep really is. Finding a way to get the right amount of high-quality sleep should be a high priority for everyone. The significance of sleep is simply not widely recognized—but it should be!

Adequate sleep is as important to our life and health as air, water, food, shelter, and relationships. Yet sleep is often one of the first cornerstones of health to be sacrificed in the name of productivity or entertainment. The negative consequences are astounding but overlooked.

Consider how you would feel if your access to food were limited and you went through every day hungry. It would result in an immediate decline in your quality of life, including impaired energy levels, mood, cognition, productivity, and general motivation. Continued deprivation would destroy your health. This is exactly what most people living in developed countries are doing to themselves in regard to sleep.

The impact of inadequate sleep on cognitive function is certain to be profound, but the evidence is just beginning to come together. It is well known that a deficiency in certain stages of sleep will impair the "consolidation," or formation, of memories.[8] These important sleep stages tend to shorten and memory consolidation tends to decline with age, and especially with AD.[13,14] Sleep apnea and diminished REM and slow-wave sleep have all been associated with impaired performance on cognitive tests, mild cognitive impairment (MCI), and dementia.[15] A remarkable study compared the levels of beta-amyloid protein in the cerebrospinal fluid (CSF, the fluid around the brain and spinal cord) of healthy people without beta-amyloid plaque in their brains with the levels of people *with* beta-amyloid plaque accumulation (pre-Alzheimer's). Interestingly, the CSF levels of beta amyloid reached a peak about six hours after waking and fell to very low levels about six hours after falling asleep. It is thought that this fluctuation reflects the brain's production of beta-amyloid protein during waking hours and the lack of beta-amyloid protein production during high-quality sleep. The subjects with pre-Alzheimer's did not show this fluctuation but instead showed steadily present levels of beta-amyloid protein in their CSF.[16] This study suggests that high-quality sleep of adequate duration is critical to balancing beta-amyloid production with clearance of it. It is likely that poor-quality sleep and circadian-rhythm dysfunction lead to continued production or inadequate clearance of beta-amyloid protein or both. These findings comport with a study showing that chronic sleep restriction in mice increases beta-amyloid levels in cerebral fluid.[17]

Correcting sleep problems so you can get good-quality sleep and getting the right amount of sleep will improve performance on cognitive tests and improve beta-amyloid processing. However, correcting sleep problems can be challenging because many abnormalities can lead to impaired sleep. A sleep study and consultation with a sleep specialist are often required to identify the exact problem. Often, however, what is needed most is an improvement in "sleep hygiene." This term refers to lifestyle, behavioral, and psychological elements that affect sleep and can be modified. (The details of sleep hygiene are enumerated below under Achieving Optimal Sleep).

In addition to common sleep disorders and problems with sleep hygiene, people with AD often have other sleep problems that are produced by the disease itself. AD patients often have impaired melatonin secretion and experience circadian-rhythm disturbances that lead to daytime sleepiness and nighttime awakenings. Key memory-forming stages of sleep are shortened as the disease progresses. Conventional AD drugs such as Donepezil have been known to cause insomnia and make existing insomnia worse.[18] As sleep quality deteriorates, so does cognitive functioning.

The great news is that melatonin, bright-light therapy (see number 2 below), and properly timed physical activity (see number 3 below) can help control circadian-rhythm disorders in people with AD.[18] Melatonin can help promote slow-wave sleep and may exert effects on several of the fundamental abnormalities leading to AD (refer to Step 5 for more details). Sunlight, light boxes, and morning exercise can help anchor the circadian rhythm from the awake side.

Achieving Optimal Sleep

Follow these rules for what to do during the day:

1. Wake up spontaneously. If at all possible, avoid using alarm clocks and waking before dawn. The body naturally wakes at the end of a sleep cycle, when it is most ready to transition into being awake.

2. Exercise! Exercising in the morning or afternoon or both helps to optimize circadian rhythms and enhances deep-stage sleep.

3. Get natural light. Exposure to sunlight (or bright full-spectrum lights) in the morning upon awakening and throughout the day helps to optimize circadian rhythms and enhance daytime energy.

4. Wake up at the same time each day (which means going to bed at the same time each night). This also optimizes the circadian rhythms and helps to prevent delays in going to sleep at night.

5. Minimize caffeine, nicotine, and other stimulants, especially after noon.

6. Address stressful or emotionally involved problems as soon as possible during the day so that they don't disrupt sleep at night.

During the evening and night, follow these rules:

1. Have a wind-down period before bed. The body and mind should begin winding down with the sun. This means not trying to finish up work demands, exercising intensely, watching action movies, or being under bright lights during the two hours before bedtime. Find something that is limited in time and tends to help you relax and get tired. A warm bath, easy yoga or stretching, breathing exercises or meditation, progressive muscle relaxation (see p. 115), listening to calming music, and light reading are examples of activities that can be incorporated into wind-down routines.

2. Keep the lights dim after dark. Light at night is considered a possible cause of cancer. Light in the blue part of the spectrum, except at extremely low intensities, suppresses melatonin secretion and interferes with good-quality sleep; light in the red wavelengths does not do this. Keeping the lights very dim and, ideally, using red lights for reading and getting up to go to the bathroom will help promote high quality sleep. Alternatively, red sunglasses can be used.

3. Avoid alcohol, nicotine, caffeine, and large meals before bedtime. All these have been shown to disrupt sleep physiology in detrimental ways.

4. Minimize electromagnetic radiation (EMR, or "electro-smog"). This type of nonionizing radiation, in unnatural form, is emitted by wireless technologies and electronics. Studies have shown that exposure to EMR at night inhibits melatonin secretion. A simple step is to unplug the wireless modem at night, and don't sleep next to (or wear) active electronic devices.

5. Keep the bedroom cool and quiet, and use the bed only for sleeping and sexual activity.

6. Keep a pencil and paper or a journal next to the bed. Record any thoughts you have overnight that you want to remember—things you just remembered that need to get done, brilliant ideas that come to you, solutions to problems, concerns that are lingering, etc. You can leave them on the paper and not on your mind. You can also use the paper or journal to record dreams immediately upon awakening, if that interests you.

7. Use progressive muscle relaxation or the mindfulness sleep-induction technique.

8. Use imagery as you fall asleep. After relaxing, take yourself on a trip to a relaxing paradise or a perfect resting spot limited only by your imagination.

9. If you find yourself lying awake in bed, don't stay there watching the clock and tossing and turning. Get out of bed and do something relaxing such as reading, listening to relaxing music, stretching, or doing breathing exercises. Or repeat part of your wind-down routine. Then return to bed for sleep. This helps to reset the mind and the body for sleep.

Example of Before-Bed Routine

8:00 p.m.   House lights dimmed or limited to red lights. Finished with TV and computer. Light reading, conversation, or music. Enjoy a cup of caffeine-free herbal tea.

9:00 p.m.   Get everything ready for bed and then enjoy a warm bath with lavender and jasmine essential oils, meditation, breathing exercises, or light stretching or yoga for thirty minutes. Keep lights very low or off.

9:45 p.m.   Lie in bed and begin progressive muscle relax-
               ation, the mindfulness sleep-induction technique,
               the use of imagery, or a combination of these.
10:00 p.m.   Sleep.

Progressive Muscle Relaxation Technique

If possible, have someone else read these steps for you or record them so you can listen to them instead of reading them.

1. Lie in bed and prepare to fall asleep.

2. Assume a passive attitude and focus on your body.

3. Tense and relax each muscle group as follows:

    a. Forehead: Wrinkle your forehead; try to make your eyebrows touch your hairline for five seconds. Relax.
    b. Eyes and nose: Close your eyes as tightly as you can for five seconds. Relax.
    c. Lips, cheeks, and jaw: Draw the centers of your mouth back and grimace for five seconds. Relax. Feel the warmth and calmness in your face.
    d. Hands: Extend your arms in front of you. Clench your fists tightly for five seconds. Relax. Feel the warmth and calmness in your hands.
    e. Forearms: Extend your arms against an invisible wall and push forward with your hands for five seconds. Relax.
    f. Upper arms: Bend your elbows and tense your biceps for five seconds. Relax. Feel the tension leave your arms.
    g. Shoulders: Shrug your shoulders up to your ears for five seconds. Relax.
    h. Back: Arch your back off the bed for five seconds. Relax. Feel the tension disappearing.
    i. Stomach: Tighten your stomach muscles for five seconds. Relax.

j. Hips and buttocks: Tighten your hip and buttock muscles for five seconds. Relax.

k. Thighs: Tighten your thigh muscles by pressing your legs together as tightly as you can for five seconds. Relax.

l. Feet: Bend your ankles toward your body as far as you can for five seconds. Relax.

m. Toes: Curl your toes as tightly as you can for five seconds. Relax.

4. Assess for remaining tense muscles. Tighten and relax those muscles four times.

5. Experience the deep relaxation of your body and the peace of your mind.

Mindfulness Sleep-Induction Technique

The following technique was adapted from a handout on integrative medicine by David Rakel, MD, of the University of Wisconsin.[19]

1. Lie in bed and prepare to fall asleep.

2. Begin with abdominal breathing: To check that you are doing abdominal breathing, place one hand on your chest and one on your abdomen. Breathe in so that the hand on the abdomen rises higher than the hand on the chest.

3. Take a slow, deep breath in through your nose for a count of 3 to 4 and exhale slowly through your mouth for a count of 6 to 7.

4. Allow your thoughts to focus on your breath and the air gently entering and leaving your nose and mouth.

5. Repeat this cycle for eight breaths.

6. After eight breaths, change your body position in bed and repeat for another eight breaths. Continue this cycle of position changes and eight breaths. It's rare to complete four cycles before falling asleep.

STEP 6: Summary of Recommendations

▶ Do brain aerobics by practicing focused cognitive activities every day.

▶ Practice mindfulness meditation.

▶ Stay connected with friends and family, meet new people, and use support groups.

▶ Follow our guidelines for pursuing high-quality sleep, and enlist the help of a sleep specialist if you need one.

❖

CLOSING NOTE FROM THE AUTHORS

Back in the Driver's Seat

The Results Depend on Your Efforts

When we first explain our Six-Step Program to new patients, some of them are understandably skeptical. They believe that Alzheimer's disease is incurable because there's no single drug or treatment that can prevent or reverse it. As a society, we've been conditioned to hope and pray for a magic bullet, but AD is far too complex for one single remedy. That's why our program has six steps and uses over thirty elements that protect and defend the brain from the root causes of AD.

The medical community's abysmal failure to prevent and treat Alzheimer's disease calls for an approach that breaks with convention and enters new territory. For this new approach to be successful, however, it must retain scientific integrity and be guided by the evidence. Fortunately, information is abundant, but no one had translated the complex concepts and results into a practical approach until now. With our approach, you honestly have nothing to lose and everything to gain.

At the Leonardi Institute, we reviewed all clinically relevant scientific research that's been done on AD and dementia over the past twenty years. While the process was painstaking, it was worth it: We identified the most powerful approaches and potent formulas and strategically combined them to produce dramatic results. We're seeing positive results with our patients, and we want the same positive results for you.

A Few Words from Our Patients

"Two weeks into this new life I find my mind is sharper and my focus stronger than ever. I'm sleeping better and rising refreshed and ready for the new day. I have been getting to work earlier and getting far more accomplished than ever."
Randy

"I entered Dr. Leonardi's program when I was sixty years old. Six months later, my husband, soul mate, and business partner of thirty-one years died suddenly, unexpectedly. During the dark days that followed, I forced myself to faithfully adhere to the program's regimen: exercise, nutrition awareness, bioidentical hormone replacement, and supplements…I am convinced that without the benefits of the program, I would not have had the energy or cognitive ability to step up as senior partner and successfully manage our design firm or to successfully manage my deceased husband's investment portfolio in addition to my own. Six weeks ago I began to learn a second language (German) via Rosetta Stone. To my delight and to my Swiss-German friends' amazement, I can now converse with them in choppy sentences…I am ecstatic—because I am sixty-six (almost). *Danke*, Dr. Dave! Without you as coach and your program, I could never have known the joy of learning another language. Italian is next."
Rosemary

"I remember names much better than I used to. For that matter, my wife used to serve as my memory bank, and now we both noticed a reversal in this role."

Peter

Getting the Support You Need to Be Successful

We're not going to sugarcoat the truth and tell you it will be a cinch to incorporate all six steps into your daily life. At first, applying the information for all six steps at the same time can be a bit complex. Don't worry. This transition period happens to everyone. But as with learning to drive a car or starting a new job, in just a few weeks or so you'll have a new routine that feels doable. And it's nothing that our prevention patients aren't already doing, including our own doctors, who are very proactive about health.

We strongly recommend that you seek the support of a doctor who is knowledgeable about AD and also ask a family member or friend to help you create a new routine that includes all six of the steps. Working with your team under the supervision of your doctor will enable you to make this comprehensive program part of your daily life.

At the Leonardi Institute, we teach people how to apply this new information to their lives. Working together with our patients, we design and administer comprehensive programs to help them accomplish their intended goals. We supply the necessary elements, and we monitor and coach our patients to ensure success.

We've been successful in reversing heart disease, diabetes, obesity, and osteoporosis. We believe our programs are also very effective in preventing many cancers. It was in applying these same principles to Alzheimer's disease that we gained our insight. Such a comprehensive and holistic approach to AD has never before been constructed.

The comprehensive treatment program for people with mild to moderate Alzheimer's disease that we use at the Leonardi Institute is the same one we offer in this book. The earlier the program is applied, the greater the likelihood of success. If you live in Colorado or have the financial means to travel here once every year or two, we'd love to be your partner in fighting this disease. If not, we sincerely hope you can find a physician nearby who, with this book as a guide, can help you to achieve the same promising results our patients are enjoying.

How the Six-Step Program Works

It's important that you understand that we are not in the practice of treating merely the symptoms of Alzheimer's disease—our goal is to arrest or reverse the disease. We are currently enrolling Alzheimer's patients in a pilot clinical trial. We're optimistic that the results these patients get will be groundbreaking and we're convinced that no other treatment is as promising based on current evidence. Our hope is to publish the results within three years, offering proof that the progression of AD can be stopped and even reversed.

At our institute, patients begin the program with extensive testing:

▶ Genetic testing to determine predisposition for Alzheimer's

▶ Screening for other potential causes of the cognitive decline

▶ Extensive cognitive testing to pinpoint the precise level of cognitive function and decline; this establishes a firm baseline so we can assess how well the program is working.

We also screen for other diseases such as cancer, heart disease, lipoprotein (cholesterol-related) problems, diabetes, prediabetes, kidney disease, and liver disease. This is a very comprehensive evaluation with abundant one-on-one time with the doctor.

Once we have reviewed all the test results and spent time getting to know our patient, we customize the Six-Step Program to his or her ability to participate, keeping disabilities and other health challenges in mind. The way we tailor each program is also dependent on the availability of the patient's caretaker. As we said earlier, following the full program correctly takes considerable effort. Therefore you will have much greater success with the supervision and coaching of your doctor and the support of your family, friends, and in some cases your caretaker.

The Six-Step Program includes the following components:
► Nutritional protocols

► Supplements

► Medications*

► Physical activities

► Mental activities

► Hormones (if indicated)

*The prescription medications in our program are not the medicines typically prescribed for Alzheimer's disease. As stated earlier, those medications merely attempt to temporarily boost memory by increasing the production of the neurotransmitter acetylcholine in the brain. Even when these medications work, the disease progresses. The medications we use target the root causes, which are the underlying biochemical processes that lead to the damage and dysfunction of AD.

Are the Benefits Worth the Effort?

You're the only one who can decide whether committing to our Six-Step Program is worth your time and effort. We've made it clear that our program is not as simple as swallowing a pill every day. For prevention, it will require some changes in your lifestyle routine. For treatment of existing cognitive impairment, both you and your caretaker will need to exert some effort. There is a drink to mix and take twice a day. There are nutritional-supplement capsules to take and one to three creams to apply to your skin each day. There is a nutritional protocol to follow as closely as possible, and we'll ask you to exercise as much as you can within your limitations. You'll also need to drop in at your local lab for a blood test three or four times a year.

If you can't come see us, don't let that discourage you. With the help of a good primary-care physician, you can certainly learn this program and follow it. He or she probably won't be familiar with this program, so you'll be responsible for much of the management. Its comprehensive nature is the reason our program is physician-supervised and why our program provides each patient with unlimited contact with our physicians for issues related to the program.

By the way, when we say a "good" physician, we mean one who will care enough about you to learn a bit about our program, prescribe the necessary hormones, monitor, and coach you. If your doctor isn't up to the task, we urge you to find one who is. If you can't find one, we sincerely hope you can make your way to Denver so we can guide you in this program every step of the way.

We share your wish that it were as simple as taking a pill or two every day, but to give yourself a fighting chance, you have to deal with the reality of this complex disease. Although it will take a little while to figure out how to smoothly incorporate all six steps and their associated thirty elements, with practice and perseverance, the program will become very manageable.

And it goes without saying that the required effort will provide a far better course than sitting back and allowing your brain to continue to deteriorate. Whether you have mild to moderate Alzheimer's disease or mild cognitive impairment, or you simply want to reduce your risk of developing either of these conditions, our Six-Step Program is your best chance of reversing, slowing, and preventing Alzheimer's disease.

We wish you the very best and
hope you've found our Six-Step Program a useful
and effective approach.

Leonardi Institute
225 Union Blvd. Suite 400
Lakewood, CO. 80228
303-462-5344
www.LeonardiInstitute.com

We also welcome your feedback and insights regarding your experience by e-mailing us at myalzheimersexperience@leonardiinstitute.com. Unfortunately, we're not able to answer specific questions submitted to this address, but the information you share will be used to determine topics for our newsletter.

To register for our free newsletter, visit us at www.LeonardiInstitute.com and click on NEWSLETTER.

The nutritional and herbal supplements discussed in this book can be found at www.Cycle-Breakers.com.

About the Authors

■ David Leonardi, MD

Dr. Leonardi is a well-known authority in vitality and longevity medicine. He is board certified in antiaging medicine, and is a Certified Nutrition Specialist and a professional member of the American Diabetes Association. A graduate of the University of Miami School of Medicine, he completed his internship in internal medicine and residency in emergency medicine at an affiliate hospital of the University of California, San Francisco. In 1986, Dr. Leonardi came to the realization that we can and must do far more for age-related disease than last-minute heroics. To that end, he left the field of emergency medicine for family and preventive medicine, and in 1997 he entered the full-time practice of vitality and longevity medicine. In 2003, he founded the Leonardi Institute, the world's most effective and evidence-based preventive medical practice in the world. This unique practice aims to generate novel approaches to disease prevention through physician-led research and the innovative synthesis of the scientific evidence.

Dr. Leonardi is in high demand as a corporate speaker. In addition to speaking at national and international physician conferences and for private corporations, he has delivered more than one hundred seminars to Vistage International and Vistage Canada, organizations of chief executive officers.

In addition, Dr. Leonardi holds four patents for medical devices that have been used in the United States for the past twenty-three years. He is an avid downhill skier and cyclist, and his passion is to continue research and development and the expansion of his programs to bring vitality and longevity medicine to the mainstream. Dr. Leonardi is happily married with two children.

■ Nathan Daley, MD, MPH

Dr. Daley is residency-trained in preventive medicine, integrative medicine, diagnostic radiology, and environmental health. In the pursuit of understanding the true entity of health, Dr. Daley has acquired an impressive background in emerging areas of medicine. After receiving an undergraduate degree in microbiology and his MD from the University of Oklahoma, Dr. Daley underwent a clinical internship and diagnostic radiology training at the Mayo Clinic in Jacksonville, Florida.

Frustrated by the overemphasis on end-stage disease and the lack of health-oriented pursuits in modern medicine, Dr. Daley began investigating the origins of health from an ecological perspective, involving gene-environment relationships and an individual's way of interacting with the environment.

An interest in complex systems science helped to frame this new understanding of health in a manageable paradigm. Encouraged that a powerful approach to optimizing health and well-being could be developed, Dr. Daley left the specialty of radiology to accumulate additional knowledge and expertise in more optimal health-oriented specialties.

Subsequently, he completed a residency in preventive medicine at the University of California, San Diego and earned a master's degree in public health in environmental health at San Diego State University. Additionally, he was one of twenty-two clinicians to be selected by the Bravewell Collaborative in 2008 as an integrative medicine fellow. This honor provided him the opportunity to receive training directly from several pioneers in integrative medicine at the University of Arizona Program in Integrative Medicine in Tucson as well as at the Scripps Center for Integrative Medicine in La Jolla, California.

Dr. Daley's clinical approach consists of partnering with his patients to develop an individualized strategy drawing from "the best of all things that work." He sees the many healing paradigms present today all as pieces of the puzzle of health, and includes himself within the emerging fields of integrative medicine, functional medicine, lifestyle medicine, and vitality and longevity medicine.

✣

WHY BIOIDENTICAL HORMONE REPLACEMENT THERAPY DURING MENOPAUSE IS SAFE

The Myth About Hormone Replacement Therapy

This myth was started in 2003 when a series of articles was published in the *Journal of the American Medical Association* presenting and interpreting results of a study called the *Women's Health Initiative* (WHI). The articles reported that hormone replacement therapy (HRT) entailed more risks and fewer benefits for most women in menopause than was previously thought. While the findings of the WHI appear to be valid, the WHI was not a study of hormone replacement therapy at all. Rather, it specifically studied two *drugs that were designed to mimic HRT*. Indeed, these *drugs* were shown to have more risks than benefits, but HRT was also incorrectly implicated as being harmful.

The problem here is not about the study results. The problem is in the ambiguous and confusing naming of the drugs that were studied. The problem began sixty years ago when researchers first began studies on estrogen replacement in postmenopausal women. At the time, there were few compounds available to replace estrogen. Regardless of the type of estrogen used, it was simply referred to as hormone replacement therapy or HRT. Unfortunately, this imprecise nomenclature stuck, and over the next six decades of medical progress, any estrogen compound used could be referred to as HRT. We now know that there are tremendous differences in the effects on our bodies' biochemistry of these various estrogenic compounds. Therefore, the term *HRT* is extremely confusing, to say the least, because it lumps all these compounds into one "class," despite their inherent and profound differences. Yet the scientific community continues to use the term with impunity—this is a travesty.

In the *Women's Health Initiative*, the HRT in question consisted of conjugated equine estrogen. Conjugated equine estrogen contains twenty-three estrogenic compounds native to horses, only two of which are native to the human body. Its origin is the urine of pregnant mares. The second drug used in the WHI was medroxyprogesterone, *a synthetic compound never produced in the human body.* It was synthesized in an effort to mimic human progesterone. So while these two drugs are referred to as HRT, *in the context of human use, they are foreign substances and not at all the hormones that are made by the human ovary.* Any rational scientist would consider such an ambiguous nomenclature unthinkable. Nonetheless, that's the way it was published. Unfortunately, referring to these two drugs as HRT leads to the implication that all hormone replacement is as hazardous as these two drugs.

If you have an illness in which a gland stops making a needed hormone, would you choose to replace the hormone precisely or would you choose instead to take a drug that mimics some of the effects of that hormone? You don't need to be a doctor to answer that question: Choosing the latter would be akin to replacing a carburetor with a brake pad.

Because of the overwhelming confusion this has caused the public, we who trust the safety of *true* hormone replacement have had to call it *bioidentical hormone replacement therapy* (BHRT) to differentiate it from drugs called HRT. The term *bioidentical* means that the hormone being used has the same molecular structure as that made by the human body. The implication for human health is vastly different.

The Science of Hormone Molecules

It's also logical that there would be a difference in the safety and efficacy of different molecules. In fact, it's none other than the molecular structure that determines the hormone's activity at specific receptor sites. If millions of years of evolution have selected the molecules and receptors in the human body, it can be concluded that the match between the two is finely tuned and purposeful. A molecule that's different from that produced by the human body in any way could logically be expected to produce a different effect from the natural (endogenous) molecule. In general, it's hard to improve the human body with modern technology, while it remains quite easy to cause harm.

The WHI: Why the Drugs Caused Problems but BHRT Does Not

The above argument explains why the negative findings in the WHI should not be attributed to bioidentical hormone replacement or any treatment other than the two drugs used in the study. However, it doesn't prove that bioidentical HRT is safe. Studies are currently underway, but we can gain significant insight into the issue if we take a look at women's adverse reactions to the two drugs in the WHI: conjugated equine estrogen and medroxyprogesterone. The reactions were largely of six types:

▶ More heart attacks

▶ More strokes

▶ More blood clots in the legs

▶ More blood clots in the lungs

▶ More dementia

▶ More breast cancer

On this list, the first five items are related to a blood clot. A heart attack is a blood clot in a coronary (heart) artery. A stroke is a blood clot in a brain artery. Blood clots in legs and lungs are self-explanatory. The type of dementia that occurred in the WHI was never determined. In our opinion, the increase was probably due not to Alzheimer's disease but to *vascular dementia*, the variety caused by clots in tiny arteries in the brain—not large enough to cause a stroke but just enough to kill a few brain cells at a time, resulting in a loss of intellect. What makes us so sure? For one thing, the dementia came on more rapidly than would be typical of Alzheimer's. More importantly, however, conjugated equine estrogen, when swallowed, causes blood clots! In fact, any estrogen causes blood clots when swallowed. Here's why: When the daily dose of estrogen is swallowed, 100 percent of the absorbed estrogen goes immediately from the intestine to the liver—just like everything else we swallow, including a hamburger. The impact of that entire daily dose of estrogen arriving at the liver all at once is to increase the liver's production of clotting proteins. The liver is where these proteins are made, and yes, estrogen accelerates that process. With more clotting proteins come more blood clots. How can we be certain about this? This physiological effect isn't even argued in the medical community, and it is taught to every medical student. It has long been known that the use of birth-control pills (which contain synthetic estrogens) increases the risk of blood clots.

It's common practice to recommend contraception other than birth control pills for women over thirty-five who smoke, because the risk of clotting is further elevated in smokers. Moreover, a study performed by some very astute investigators in England confirmed this effect of oral estrogen. It was published in England's most prestigious medical journal, *The Lancet*. In the study, postmenopausal women were assigned to receive one of three treatments: oral estrogen, transdermal estrogen (applied to the skin), or a placebo. The doses were adjusted so that the blood level of estrogen was the same between the orally dosed group and the skin-cream group. While the women given oral estrogen experienced three and a half times more blood clots than those on the placebo, those given transdermal estrogen actually had 10 percent *fewer* blood clots than the placebo group.[1]

Why doesn't bioidentical human estrogen applied to the skin cause blood clots? Because it's not swallowed. Rather than going to the liver all at once from the intestine, it enters the general circulation through the skin, just like estrogen made by the human ovary enters the general circulation from the ovary. The liver, then, only receives its very small share, and gradually, causing no effect on clotting proteins. The moral of this story is that estrogen should never be swallowed. This is why at the Leonardi Institute *we provide only bioidentical HRT and never provide estrogen by mouth.* We administer estrogen only in a transdermal cream, which is absorbed and distributed throughout the body evenly, just as if it were being made by the ovary.

The above discussion covers all the adverse events seen in the WHI except breast cancer. It was anticipated in the WHI that breast cancer would be slightly more common in women on conjugated equine estrogen than those on a placebo because estrogen is a breast stimulant no matter how it's given. But we don't know if bioidentical HRT increases breast-cancer risk. Actually, early studies have suggested that bioidentical estradiol and progesterone, used together, may *reduce* breast-cancer risk.[2] However, more studies are needed to confirm this. Therefore, we employ a nutritional supplement that we believe, when used as part of our comprehensive approach to health optimization, effectively neutralizes any increased risk of breast cancer inherent in BHRT. There are actually two such supplements, and both work the same way. One is a vegetable compound called indole-3-carbinol (I3C), and the other is an active byproduct of the same compound called diindolylmethane (or DIM for short). They both come from cruciferous vegetables (broccoli, cauliflower, cabbage, brussels sprouts, bok choy, and kale). It's relevant to note here that higher intakes of cruciferous vegetables have been associated with lower rates of breast cancer in epidemiologic studies.[3] These nutritional supplements work by altering the metabolic pathway of estradiol in the human body. Estradiol is the most prominent estrogen made by the human ovary. Normally, estradiol is broken down into three byproducts. Two have been demonstrated to be cancer-promoting to the breast; the third is harmless. I3C and DIM promote the conversion of estradiol into the third (harmless) byproduct and eliminate much of the two cancer-promoting byproducts. The result is a dramatically reduced risk of breast cancer.

Using these compounds and several other natural techniques for cancer prevention, we have seen only one case of breast cancer in our entire practice in the past thirteen years. Here's an important concept illustrated by our track record on breast cancer: It's *normal* for women to make these two cancer-promoting estrogens, and it's *normal* for a significant percentage of women to develop breast cancer. It's the most common cancer in women and is responsible for more cancer deaths than any other. What we do is perform constant research to find all the nutritional compounds and lifestyle habits we can to help people move from *normal* to *optimal*. Our programs demonstrate significant success in the prevention of heart disease, cancer, obesity, diabetes, osteoporosis, and, yes, Alzheimer's disease. The use of bioidentical HRT and the use of DIM or indole-3-carbinol are two of our techniques.

References

References for Step 1: "Rustproofing"

1. W. R. Markesbery, "Oxidative Stress Hypothesis in Alzheimer's Disease," *Free Radical Biology & Medicine* 23, no. 1 (1997): 134–47.

2. L. T. McGrath et al., "Increased Oxidative Stress In Alzheimer's Disease as Assessed with 4-hydroxynonenal but not Malondialdehyde," *Monthly Journal of the Association of Physicians* 94, no. 9 (2001): 485–90.

3. M. R. Prasad et al., "Regional Membrane Phospholipid Alterations in Alzheimer's Disease," *Neurochemistry Research* 23, no. 1 (2001): 81–8.

4. J. W. Jama et al., "Dietary Antioxidants and Cognitive Function in a Population-Based Sample of Older Persons: The Rotterdam Study," *American Journal of Epidemiology* 144, no. 3 (1996): 275–80.

5. A. Skoumalova et al., "The Role of Free Radicals in Canine Counterpart of Senile Dementia of the Alzheimer Type," *Experimental Gerontology* 38, no. 6 (2003): 711–9.

6. B. L. Sopher et al., "Neurodegenerative Mechanisms in Alzheimer Disease: A Role for Oxidative Damage in Amyloid Beta Protein Precursor-Mediated Cell Death," *Molecular and Chemical Neuropathology* 29, no. 2–3 (1996): 153–68.

7. M. A. Pappolla et al., "Melatonin Prevents Death of Neuroblastoma Cells Exposed to the Alzheimer Amyloid Peptide," *The Journal of Neuroscience* 17, no. 5 (1997): 1683–90.

8. M. A. Pappolla et al., "Evidence of Oxidative Stress and In Vivo Neurotoxicity of Beta-Amyloid in a Transgenic Mouse Model of Alzheimer's Disease: A Chronic Oxidative Paradigm for Testing Antioxidant Therapies In Vivo," *The American Journal of Pathology* 152, no. 4 (1998): 871–7.

9. R. J. Mark et al., "Basic FGF Attenuates Amyloid Beta-Peptide-Induced Oxidative Stress, Mitochondrial Dysfunction, and Impairment of Na+/K+-ATPase Activity in Hippocampal Neurons." *Brain Research* 756, no. 1–2 (1997): 205–14.

10. C. Behl and F. Holsboer, ["Oxidative Stress in the Pathogenesis of Alzheimer's Disease and Antioxidant Neuroprotection,"] *Fortschritte der Neurologie-Psychiatrie* 66, no. 3 (1998): 113–21. [in German].

11. D. Paris et al., "Role of Peroxynitrite in the Vasoactive and Cytotoxic Effects of Alzheimer's Beta-Amyloid 1-40 Peptide," *Experimental Neurology* 152, no. 1 (1998): 116–22.

12. D. W. Molloy et al., "Effects of Acute Exposure to Aluminum on Cognition in Humans," *Journal of Toxicology and Environmental Health Part A* 70, no. 23 (2007): 2011–9.

13. D. R. Crapper McLachlan et al., "Intramuscular Desferrioxamine in Patients with Alzheimer's Disease," *The Lancet* 337, no. 8753 (1991): 1304–8. [Erratum. *Lancet* 337, no. 8757 (1991): 1618.]

14. D. R. McLachlan, P. E. Fraser, and A. J. Dalton, "Aluminium and the Pathogenesis of Alzheimer's Disease: A Summary of Evidence," *Ciba Foundation Symposium* 169 (1992): 87–98. Discussion. 99–108.

15. D. R. McLachlan, W. L. Smith, and T. P. Kruck, "Desferrioxamine and Alzheimer's Disease: Video Home Behavior Assessment of Clinical Course and Measures of Brain Aluminum," *Therapeutic Drug Monitoring* 15, no. 6 (1993): 602–7.

16. G. A. Taylor et al., "Alzheimer's Disease and the Relationship Between Silicon and Aluminium in Water Supplies in Northern England," *Journal of Epidemiology and Community Health* 49, no. 3 (1995): 323–4.

17. W. F. Forbes and J. F. Gentleman, "Risk Factors, Causality, and Policy Initiatives: The Case of Aluminum and Mental Impairment," *Experimental Gerontology* 33, no. 1–2 (1998): 141–54.

18. G. F. Van Landeghem et al., "Transferrin C2, Metal Binding and Alzheimer's Disease," *Neuroreport* 9, no. 2 (1998): 177–9.

19. P. B. Moore, "Absorption of Aluminium-26 in Alzheimer's Disease, Measured Using Accelerator Mass Spectrometry," *Dementia and Geriatric Cognitive Disorders* 11, no. 2 (2000): 66–9.

20. C. Exley et al., "Non-Invasive Therapy to Reduce the Body Burden of Aluminium in Alzheimer's Disease," *Journal of Alzheimer's Disease* 10, no. 1 (2006): 17–24. Discussion. 29–31.

21. L. Gerhardsson et al., "Metal Concentrations in Plasma and Cerebrospinal Fluid in Patients with Alzheimer's Disease," *Dementia and Geriatric Cognitive Disorders* 25, no. 6 (2008): 508–15.

22. J. Mutter et al., ["Mercury and Alzheimer's Disease,"]. *Fortschritte der Neurologie-Psychiatrie* 75, no. 9 (2007): 528–38. [in German].

23. R. A. Yokel, "Blood-Brain Barrier Flux of Aluminum, Manganese, Iron and Other Metals Suspected to Contribute to Metal-Induced Neurodegeneration," *Journal of Alzheimer's Disease* 10, no. 2–3 (2006): 223–53.

24. C. Hock et al., "Increased Blood Mercury Levels in Patients with Alzheimer's Disease," *Journal of Neural Transmission* 105, no. 1 (1998): 59–68.

25. C. C. Leong, N. I. Syed, and F. L. Lorscheider, "Retrograde Degeneration of Neurite Membrane Structural Integrity of Nerve Growth Cones Following In Vitro Exposure to Mercury," *Neuroreport* 12, no. 4 (2001): 733–7.

26. S. Bucossi et al., "Copper in Alzheimer's Disease: A Meta-Analysis of Serum, Plasma, and Cerebrospinal Fluid Studies," *Journal of Alzheimer's Disease* 24, no. 1 (2011): 175–85.

27. J. F. Quinn et al., "A Copper-Lowering Strategy Attenuates Amyloid Pathology in a Transgenic Mouse Model of Alzheimer's Disease," *Journal of Alzheimer's Disease* 21, no. 3 (2010): 903–14.

28. G. J. Brewer et al., "Copper and Ceruloplasmin Abnormalities in Alzheimer's Disease," *American Journal of Alzheimer's Disease and Other Dementias* 25, no. 6 (2010): 490–7.

29. Z. Zheng et al., "Altered Microglial Copper Homeostasis in a Mouse Model of Alzheimer's Disease, "*Journal of Neurochemistry* 114, no. 6 (2010): 1630–8.

30. G. J. Brewer, "The Risks of Copper Toxicity Contributing to Cognitive Decline in the Aging Population and to Alzheimer's Disease," *Journal of the American College of Nutrition* 28, no. 3 (2009): 238–42.

31. R. Squitti and C. Salustri, "Agents Complexing Copper as a Therapeutic Strategy for the Treatment of Alzheimer's Disease," *Current Alzheimer Research* 6, no. 6 (2009): 476–87.

32. J. R. Walton, "A Longitudinal Study of Rats Chronically Exposed to Aluminum at Human Dietary Levels," *Neuroscience Letters* 412, no. 1 (2007): 29–33.

33. S. M. Saiyed and R. A. Yokel. "Aluminium Content of Some Foods and Food Products in the USA, with Aluminium Food Additives," *Food Additives and Contaminants* 22, no. 3 (2005): 234–44.

34. B. Liu et al., "Iron Promotes the Toxicity of Amyloid Beta Peptide by Impeding its Ordered Aggregation," *The Journal of Biological Chemistry* 286, no. 6 (2011) 4248–56.

35. X. Li, J. Jankovic, and W. Le. "Iron Chelation and Neuroprotection in Neurodegenerative Diseases," *Journal of Neural Transmission* 118, no. 3 (2011): 473–7.

36. A. C. Leskovjan et al., "Increased Brain Iron Coincides with Early Plaque Formation in a Mouse Model of Alzheimer's Disease," *Neuroimage* 55, no. 1 (2011): 32–8.

37. S. Bandyopadhyay et al., "Novel Drug Targets Based on Metallobiology of Alzheimer's Disease," *Expert Opinion on Therapeutic Targets* 14, no. 11 (2010): 1177–97.

38. D. B. Kell, "Towards a Unifying, Systems Biology Understanding of Large-Scale Cellular Death and Destruction Caused by Poorly Liganded Iron: Parkinson's, Huntington's, Alzheimer's, Prions, Bactericides, Chemical Toxicology and Others as Examples," *Archives of Toxicology* 84, no. 11 (2010): 825–89.

39. T. S. Anekonda et al., "Phytic Acid as a Potential Treatment of Alzheimer's Pathology: Evidence from Animal and In

Vitro Models," *Journal of Alzheimer's Disease* 23, no. 1 (2011): 21–35.

40. L. F. Jiang et al., "Impacts of Cd(II) on the Conformation and Self-Aggregation of Alzheimer's Tau Fragment Corresponding to the Third Repeat of Microtubule-Binding Domain," *Biochimica et Biophysica Acta* 1774, no. 11 (2007): 1414–21.

41. H. Gu et al., 2011. "Lead Exposure Increases Levels of β-amyloid in the Brain and CSF and Inhibits LRP1 Expression in APP Transgenic Mice," *Neuroscience Letters* 490, no. 1 (2011): 16–20.

42. N. Li et al., "Increased Tau Phosphorylation and Beta Amyloid in the Hipocampus [sic] of Mouse Pups by Early Life Lead Exposure," *Acta Biologica Hungarica* 61, no. 2 (2010): 123–34.

43. M. Behl et al., "Lead-Induced Accumulation of Beta-Amyloid in the Choroid Plexus: Role of Low Density Lipoprotein Receptor Protein-1 and Protein Kinase C," *Neurotoxicology* 31, no. 5 (2010): 524–32.

44. M. Behl, Y. Zhang, and W. Zheng. "Involvement of Insulin-Degrading Enzyme in the Clearance of Beta-Amyloid at the Blood-CSF Barrier: Consequences of Lead Exposure," *Cerebrospinal Fluid Research* 6 (2009): 11.

45. F. Grases et al., "Dietary Phytate and Mineral Bioavailability," *Journal of Trace Elements in Medicine and Biology* 15, no. 4 (2001): 221–8.

46. S. Ou, K. Gao, and Y. Li. "An In Vitro Study of Wheat Bran Binding Capacity of Hg, Cd, and Pb," *Journal of Agricultural and Food Chemistry* 47, no. 11 (1999): 4714–7.

47. N. T. Davies and R. Nightingale. "The Effects of Phytate on Intestinal Absorption and Secretion of Zinc, and Whole-Body Retention of Zn, Copper, Iron and Manganese in

Rats," *The British Journal of Nutrition* 34, no. 2 (1975): 243–58.

48. A. M. García, A. Sisternas, and S. P. Hoyos. "Occupational Exposure to Extremely Low Frequency Electric and Magnetic Fields and Alzheimer Disease: A Meta-Analysis," *International Journal of Epidemiology* 37, no. 2 (2008): 329–40.

49. D. Carpenter and C. Sage, editors. August 31, 2007. "BioInitiative Report: A Rationale for a Biologically-Based Public Exposure Standard for Electromagnetic Fields (ELF and RF)." *BioInitiative.* http://www.bioinitiative.org/freeaccess/report/docs/report.pdf. (Accessed January 17, 2012.)

References for Step 2: Prevent "Sticky" Protein Cells

1. A. M. Schmidt et al., "Receptor for Advanced Glycation End Products (AGEs) Has a Central Role in Vessel Wall Interactions and Gene Activation in Response to Circulating AGE Proteins," *Proceedings of the National Academy of Sciences of the United States of America* 91, no. 19 (1994): 8807–11.

2. T. M. Wolever and J. B. Miller. "Sugars and Blood Glucose Control," *The American Journal of Clinical Nutrition* 62, no. 1 Suppl. (1995): 212S–221S. Discussion. 221S–7S.

3. J. A. Luchsinger, "Adiposity, Hyperinsulinemia, Diabetes and Alzheimer's Disease: An Epidemiological Perspective," *European Journal of Pharmacology* 585, no. 1 (2008): 119–29.

4. L. D. Baker et al., "Effects of Aerobic Exercise on Mild Cognitive Impairment: A Controlled Trial," *Archives of Neurology* 67, no. 1 (2010): 71–9.

5. N. T. Lautenschlager et al., "Effect of Physical Activity on Cognitive Function in Older Adults at Risk for Alzheimer Disease: A Randomized Trial," *The Journal of the American Medical Association* 300, no. 9 (2008): 1027–37.

6. E. Santana-Sosa et al., "Exercise Training is Beneficial for Alzheimer's Patients," *International Journal of Sports Medicine* 29, no. 10 (2008): 845–50.

7. C. L. Williams and R. M. Tappen, "Exercise Training for Depressed Older Adults with Alzheimer's Disease," *Aging & Mental Health* 12, no. 1 (2008): 72–80.

8. Y. S. Kwak et al., "Effect of Regular Exercise on Senile Dementia Patients," *International Journal of Sports Medicine* 29, no. 6 (2008): 471–4.

9. M. Krause and J. C. Rodrigues-Krause, "Extracellular Heat Shock Proteins (eHSP70) in Exercise: Possible Targets Outside the Immune System and Their Role for Neurodegenerative Disorders Treatment," *Medical Hypotheses* 76, no. 2 (2011): 286–90.

10. A. M. Stranahan et al., "Pharmacomimetics of Exercise: Novel Approaches for Hippocampally-Targeted Neuroprotective Agents," *Current Medicinal Chemistry* 16, no. 35 (2009): 4668–78.

References for Step 3: Make Your Genes Work in Your Favor

1. J. A. Lemon, D. R. Boreham, and C. D. Rollo, "A Dietary Supplement Abolishes Age-Related Cognitive Decline in Transgenic Mice Expressing Elevated Free Radical Processes," *Experimental Biology and Medicine* (*Maywood, N.J.*) 228, no. 7 (2003): 800–10.

2. J. A. Lemon, D. R. Boreham, and C. D. Rollo, *The Journals of Gerontology Series A, Biological Sciences and Medical Sciences* 60, no. 3 (2005): 275–9.

3. J. A. Lemon, C. D. Rollo, and D. R. Boreham, "Elevated DNA Damage in a Mouse Model of Oxidative Stress: Impacts of Ionizing Radiation and a Protective Dietary Supplement," *Mutagenesis* 23, no. 6 (2008): 473–82.

4. J. A. Lemon et al., "Radiation-Induced Apoptosis in Mouse Lymphocytes is Modified by a Complex Dietary Supplement: The Effect of Genotype and Gender," *Mutagenesis* 23, no. 6 (2008): 465–72.

5. V. Aksenov et al., "Dietary Amelioration of Locomotor, Neurotransmitter and Mitochondrial Aging," *Experimental Biology and Medicine (Maywood, N.J.)* 235, no. 1 (2010): 66–76.

References for Step 4: Combat the Root Causes of Alzheimer's Disease

1. L. J. Thal et al., "A 1-Year Multicenter Placebo-Controlled Study of Acetyl-L-Carnitine in Patients with Alzheimer's Disease," *Neurology* 47, no. 3 (1996): 705–11.

2. J. O. Brooks et al., 3rd, "Acetyl L-Carnitine Slows Decline in Younger Patients with Alzheimer's Disease: A Reanalysis of a Double-Blind, Placebo-Controlled Study Using the Trilinear Approach," *International Psychogeriatrics* 10, no. 2 (1998): 193–203.

3. G. Salvioli and M. Neri. "L-Acetylcarnitine Treatment of Mental Decline in the Elderly," *Drugs Under Experimental and Clinical Research* 20, no. 4 (1994): 169–76.

4. M. Sano et al., "Double-Blind Parallel Design Pilot Study of Acetyl Levocarnitine in Patients with Alzheimer's Disease," *Archives of Neurology* 49, no. 11 (1992): 1137–41.

5. A. Spagnoli et al., "Long-Term Acetyl-L-Carnitine Treatment in Alzheimer's Disease," *Neurology* 41, no. 11 (1991): 1726–32.

6. C. Cipolli and G. Chiari, ["Effects of L-Acetylcarnitine on Mental Deterioration in the Aged: Initial Results,"]. *La Clinica Terapeutica* 132, no. 6 Suppl. (1990): 479–510. [in Italian].

7. W. M. Herrmann, B. Dietrich, and R. Hiersemenzel. "Pharmaco-Electroencephalographic and Clinical Effects of the Cholinergic Substance—Acetyl-L-Carnitine—in Patients with Organic Brain Syndrome," *International Journal of Clinical Pharmacology Research* 10, 1–2 (1990): 81–4.

8. H. M. Abdul et al., Acetyl-L-Carnitine-Induced Up-Regulation of Heat Shock Proteins Protects Cortical Neurons against Amyloid-Beta Peptide 1-42-Mediated Oxidative Stress and Neurotoxicity: Implications for Alzheimer's Disease," *Journal of Neuroscience Research* 84, no. 2 (2006): 398–408.

9. G. Traina et al., "In the Rat Brain Acetyl-L-Carnitine Treatment Modulates the Expression of Genes Involved in Neuronal Ceroid Lipofuscinosis," *Molecular Neurobiology* 38, no. 2 (2008): 146–52.

10. G. Traina, G. Federighi, and M. Brunelli, "Up-Regulation of Kinesin Light-Chain 1 Gene Expression by Acetyl-L-Carnitine: Therapeutic Possibility in Alzheimer's Disease," *Neurochemistry International* 53, no. 6–8 (2008): 244–7.

11. R. Epis et al., "Modulatory Effect of Acetyl-L-Carnitine on Amyloid Precursor Protein Metabolism in Hippocampal Neurons," *European Journal of Pharmacology* 597, no. 1–3 (2008): 51–6.

12. J. Suchy, A. Chan, and T. B. Shea, "Dietary Supplementation with a Combination of Alpha-Lipoic Acid, Acetyl-L-Carnitine, Glycerophosphocoline, Docosahexaenoic Acid, and Phosphatidylserine Reduces Oxidative Damage to Murine Brain and Improves Cognitive Performance," *Nutrition Research* 29, no. 1 (2009): 70–4.

13. G. Traina et al., "Cytoprotective Effect of Acetyl-L-Carnitine Evidenced by Analysis of Gene Expression in the Rat Brain," *Molecular Neurobiology* 39, no. 2 (2009): 101–6.

14. J. C. Shenk et al., "The Effect of Acetyl-L-Carnitine and R-Alpha-Lipoic Acid Treatment in ApoE4 Mouse as a Model of Human Alzheimer's Disease," *Journal of the Neurological Sciences* 283, no. 1–2 (2009): 199–206.

15. Y. Y. Yin et al., "Acetyl-L-Carnitine Attenuates Okadaic Acid Induced Tau Hyperphosphorylation and Spatial Memory Impairment in Rats," *Journal of Alzheimer's Disease* 19, no. 2 (2010): 735–46.

16. K. Hager et al., "Alpha-Lipoic Acid as a New Treatment Option for Alzheimer [corrected] Type Dementia," *Archives of Gerontology and Geriatrics* 32, no. 3 (2001): 275–82. [Erratum. *Archives of Gerontology and Geriatrics* 51, no. 1 (2010): 110.]

17. K. Hager et al., "Alpha-Lipoic Acid as a New Treatment Option for Alzheimer's Disease: A 48 Months Follow-Up Analysis," *Journal of Neural Transmission Supplementum* 72 (): 189–93.

18. J. Gasic-Milenkovic, C. Loske, and G. Münch, "Advanced Glycation Endproducts Cause Lipid Peroxidation in the Human Neuronal Cell Line SH-SY5Y," *Journal of Alzheimer's Disease* 5, no. 1 (2003): 25–30.

19. L. Zhang et al., "Alpha-Lipoic Acid Protects Rat Cortical Neurons against Cell Death Induced My Amyloid and

Hydrogen Peroxide through the Akt Signalling Pathway," *Neuroscience Letters* 312, no. 3 (2001): 125–8.

20. W. Deuther-Conrad et al., "Advanced Glycation Endproducts Change Glutathione Redox Status in SH-SY5Y Human Neuroblastoma Cells by a Hydrogen Peroxide Dependent Mechanism," *Neuroscience Letters* 312, no. 1 (2001): 29–32.

21. M. Sharma and Y. K. Gupta. "Effect of Alpha Lipoic Acid on Intracerebroventricular Streptozotocin Model of Cognitive Impairment in Rats," *European Neuropsychopharmacology* 13, no. 4 (2003): 241–7.

22. K. Maiese et al., "The Vitamin Nicotinamide: Translating Nutrition into Clinical Care," *Molecules* 14, no. 9 (2009): 3446–85.

23. N. Braidy, G. Guillemin, and R. Grant. "Promotion of Cellular NAD(+) Anabolism: Therapeutic Potential for Oxidative Stress in Ageing and Alzheimer's Disease," *Neurotoxicity Research* 13, no. 3–4 (2008): 173–84.

24. D. Liu et al., "Nicotinamide Prevents NAD+ Depletion and Protects Neurons against Excitotoxicity and Cerebral Ischemia: NAD+ Consumption by SIRT1 May Endanger Energetically Compromised Neurons," *Neuromolecular Medicine* 11, no. 1 (2009): 28–42.

25. R. Clarke et al., "Folate, Vitamin B12, and Serum Total Homocysteine Levels in Confirmed Alzheimer Disease," *Archives of Neurology* 55, no. 11 (1998): 1449–55.

26. S. Seshadri et al., "Plasma Homocysteine as a Risk Factor for Dementia and Alzheimer's Disease," *The New England Journal of Medicine* 346, no. 7 (2002): 476–83.

27. S. P. McIlroy et al., "Moderately Elevated Plasma Homocysteine, Methylenetetrahydrofolate Reductase Genotype, and Risk for Stroke, Vascular Dementia, and

Alzheimer Disease in Northern Ireland," *Stroke* 33, no. 10 (2002): 2351–6.

28. B. Hooshmand et al., "Homocysteine and Holotranscobalamin and the Risk of Alzheimer Disease: A Longitudinal Study," *Neurology* 75, no. 16 (2010): 1408–14.

29. I. I. Kruman et al., "Folic Acid Deficiency and Homocysteine Impair DNA Repair in Hippocampal Neurons and Sensitize Them to Amyloid Toxicity in Experimental Models of Alzheimer's Disease," *The Journal of Neuroscience* 22, no. 5 (2002): 1752–62.

30. I. I. Kruman et al., "Homocysteine Elicits a DNA Damage Response in Neurons that Promotes Apoptosis and Hypersensitivity to Excitotoxicity," *The Journal of Neuroscience* 20, no. 18 (2000): 6920–6.

31. J. A. McMahon et al., "A Controlled Trial of Homocysteine Lowering and Cognitive Performance," *The New England Journal of Medicine* 354, no. 26 (2006): 2764–72.

32. J. G. van Uffelen et al., "The Effect of Walking and Vitamin B Supplementation on Quality of Life in Community-Dwelling Adults with Mild Cognitive Impairment: A Randomized, Controlled Trial," *Quality of Life Research* 16, no. 7 (2007): 1137–46.

33. K. Nilsson, L. Gustafson, and B. Hultberg, "Improvement of Cognitive Functions after Cobalamin/Folate Supplementation in Elderly Patients with Dementia and Elevated Plasma Homocysteine," *International Journal of Geriatric Psychiatry* 16, no. 6 (2001): 609–14.

34. D. S. Wald, A. Kasturiratne, and M. Simmonds, "Serum Homocysteine and Dementia: Meta-Analysis of Eight Cohort Studies Include 8669 Participants," *Alzheimer's & Dementia* 7, no. 4 (2011): 412–7.

35. M. Slomka, E. Zieminska, and J. Lazarewicz, 2008. "Nicotinamide and 1-Methylnicotinamide Reduce Homocysteine Neurotoxicity in Primary Cultures of Rat Cerebellar Granule Cells," *Acta Neurobiologiae Experimentalis* (*Warsaw*) 68 (1): 1–9.

36. K. N. Green et al., "Nicotinamide Restores Cognition in Alzheimer's Disease Transgenic Mice via a Mechanism Involving Sirtuin Inhibition and Selective Reduction of Thr231-Phosphotau," *Journal of Euroscience* 28, no. 45 (2008): 11500–10.

37. M. H. Eskelinen et al., "Midlife Coffee and Tea Drinking and the Risk of Late-Life Dementia: A Population-Based CAIDE Study," *Journal of Alzheimer's Disease* 16, no. 1 (2009): 85–91.

38. L. Maia and A. de Mendonça, "Does Caffeine Intake Protect from Alzheimer's Disease?" *European Journal of Neurology* 9, no. 4 (2002): 377–82.

39. G. W. Arendash et al., "Caffeine Protects Alzheimer's mice against Cognitive Impairment and Reduces Brain Beta-Amyloid Production," *Neuroscience* 142, no. 4 (2006): 941–52.

40. G. W. Arendash et al., "Caffeine Reverses Cognitive Impairment and Decreases Brain Amyloid-Beta Levels in Aged Alzheimer's Disease Mice," *Journal of Alzheimer's Disease* 17, no. 3 (2009): 661–80.

41. G. W. Arendash and C. Cao, "Caffeine and Coffee as Therapeutics against Alzheimer's Disease," *Journal of Alzheimer's Disease* 20, no. Suppl. 1 (2010): S117–26.

42. C. Santos et al., "Caffeine Intake is Associated with a Lower Risk of Cognitive Decline: A Cohort Study from Portugal," *Journal of Alzheimer's Disease* 20, no. Suppl. 1 (2010): S175–85.

43. K. Ritchie et al., "The Neuroprotective Effects of Caffeine: A Prospective Population Study (the Three City Study)," *Neurology* 69, no. 6 (2007): 536–45.

44. B. M. van Gelder et al., "Coffee Consumption is Inversely Associated with Cognitive Decline in Elderly European Men: The FINE Study," *European Journal of Clinical Nutrition* 61, no. 2 (2007): 226–32.

45. R. R. McCusker, B. A. Goldberger, and E. J. Cone, "Caffeine Content of Specialty Coffees," *Journal of Analytical Toxicology* 27, no. 7 (2003): 520–2.

46. M. Ganguli et al., "Apolipoprotein E Polymorphism and Alzheimer Disease: The Indo-US Cross-National Dementia Study," *Archives of Neurology* 57 (2000): 824–30.

47. Q. Y. Wei et al., "Inhibition of Lipid Peroxidation and Protein Oxidation in Rat Liver Mitochondria by Curcumin and its Analogues," *Biochemica et Biophysica Acta* 1760 (2006): 70–7.

48. S. K. Sandur et al., "Role of Pro-Oxidants and Antioxidants in the Anti-Inflammatory and Apoptotic Effects of Curcumin (Diferuloylmethane)," *Free Radical Biology & Medicine* 43, no. 4 (2007): 568–80.

49. L. Baum and A. Ng. "Curcumin Interaction with Copper and Iron Suggests One Possible Mechanism of Action in Alzheimer's Disease Animal Models," *Journal of Alzheimer's Disease* 6 (2004): 367–77. Discussion. 443–9.

50. M. L. Hegde et al., "Challenges Associated with Metal Chelation Therapy in Alzheimer's Disease," *Journal of Alzheimer's Disease* 17, no. 3 (2009): 457–68.

51. K. Ono et al., "Curcumin has Potent Anti-Amyloidogenic Effects of Alzheimer's Beta-Amyloid Fibrils In Vitro," *Journal of Neuroscience Research* 75 (2004): 742–50.

52. G. P. Lim et al., "The Curry Spice Curcumin Reduces Oxidative Damage and Amyloid Pathology in an Alzheimer Transgenic Mouse," *The Journal of Neuroscience* 21 (2001): 8370–7.

53. T. Ishrat et al., "Amelioration of Cognitive Deficits and Neurodegeneration by Curcumin in Rat Model of Sporadic Dementia of Alzheimer's type (SDAT)," *European Neuropsychopharmacology* 19 (2009): 636–47.

54. L. Zhang et al., "Curcuminoids Enhance Amyloid-Beta Uptake by Macrophages of Alzheimer's Disease Patients," *Journal of Alzheimer's Disease* 10, no. 1 (2006): 1–7.

55. A. Masoumi et al., "1alpha,25-dihydroxyvitamin D3 Interacts with Curcuminoids to Stimulate Amyloid-Beta Clearance by Macrophages of Alzheimer's Disease Patients," *Journal of Alzheimer's Disease* 17, no. 3 (2009): 703–17.

56. S. Sakai et al., "Inhibitory Effect of Ferulic Acid on Macrophage Inflammatory Protein-2 Production a Murine Macrophage In Cell Line," RAW264.7," *Cytokine* 9, no. 4 (1997): 242–8.

57. R. Sultana et al., "Ferulic Acid Ethyl Ester Protects Neurons against Amyloid Beta-Peptide(1-42)-Induced Oxidative Stress and Neurotoxicity: Relationship to Antioxidant Activity," *Journal of Neurochemistry* 92, no. 4 (2005): 749–58.

58. J. Y. Cho et al., "Inhibitory Effects of Long-Term Administration of Ferulic Acid on Astrocyte Activation Induced by Intracerebroventricular Injection of Beta-Amyloid Peptide (1-42) in Mice," *Progress in Neuro-psychopharmacology & Biological Psychiatry* 29, no. 6 (2005): 901–7.

59. Y. Jin et al., "Sodium Ferulate Prevents Amyloid-Beta-Induced Neurotoxicity through Suppression of p38 MAPK and Upregulation of ERK-1/2 and Akt/Protein Kinase B in

Rat Hippocampus," *Acta Pharmacologica Sinica* 26, no. 8 (2005): 943–51.

60. P. Picone et al., "Ferulic Acid Inhibits Oxidative Stress and Cell Death Induced by Ab Oligomers: Improved Delivery by Solid Lipid Nanoparticles," *Free Radical Research* 43, no. 11 (2009): 1133–45.

61. P. Quist-Paulsen, "Statins and Inflammation: An Update," *Current Opinion in Cardiology* 25, no. 4 (2010): 399–405.

62. B. H. Ali et al., "Some Phytochemical, Pharmacological and Toxicological Properties of Ginger (Zingiber Officinale Roscoe): A Review of Recent Research," *Food and Chemical Toxicology* 46, no. 2 (2008): 409–20.

63. M. Thomson et al., "The Use of Ginger (Zingiber Officinale Rosc.) As a Potential Anti-Inflammatory and Antithrombotic Agent," *Prostaglandins, Leukotrienes, and Essential Fatty Acids* 67 (2002): 475–8.

64. R. Grzanna et al., "Ginger Extract Inhibits Beta-Amyloid Peptide-Induced Cytokine and Chemokine Expression in Cultured THP-1 Monocytes," *Journal of Alternative and Complementary Medicine* 10, no. 6 (2004): 1009–13.

65. D. S. Kim, J. Y. Kim, and Y. S. Han. "Alzheimer's Disease Drug Discovery from Herbs: Neuroprotectivity from Beta-Amyloid (1-42) Insult," *Journal of Alternative and Complementary Medicine* 13, no. 3 (2007): 333–44.

66. M. N. Ghayur et al., "Muscarinic, Ca^{++} Antagonist and Specific Butyrylcholinesterase Inhibitory Activity of Dried Ginger Extract Might Explain Its Use in Dementia," *The Journal of Pharmacy and Pharmacology* 60, no. 10 (2008): 1375–83.

67. V. Vuksan, "American Ginseng (*Panax Quinquefolius* L.) Reduces Postprandial Glycemia in Nondiabetic Subjects

and Subjects with Type 2 Diabetes Mellitus," *Archives of Internal Medicine* 160 (2000): 1009–13.

68. G. N. Predy et al., "Efficacy of an Extract of North American Ginseng Containing Poly-Furanosyl-Pyranosyl-Saccharides for Preventing Upper Respiratory Tract Infections: A Randomized Controlled Trial," *Canadian Medical Association Journal* 173 (2005): 1043–8.

69. C. G. Benishin et al., "Effects of Ginsenoside Rb1 on Central Cholinergic Metabolism," *Pharmacology* 42 (1991): 223–9.

70. L. C. Wang et al., "Effects of Ginseng Saponins on Beta-Amyloid-Induced Amnesia in Rats," *Journal of Ethnopharmacology* 103, no. 1 (2006): 103–8.

71. S. T. Kim et al., "Neuroprotective Effect of Some Plant Extracts in Cultured CT105-Induced PC12 Cells," *Biological & Pharmaceutical Bulletin* 29, no. 10 (2006): 2021–4.

72. S. Q. Hu et al., ["Neuroprotective Effects of Water Extracts of American Ginseng on SH-SY5Y Cells Apoptosis Induced by Abeta25-35,"]. *Zhong Yao Cai* 31, no. 9 (2008): 1373–7. [in Chinese].

73. R. Zhao et al., "Implication of Phosphaitdylinositol-3 Kinase/Akt/Glycogen Synthase Kinase-3β Pathway in Ginsenoside Rb1's Attenuation of Beta-Amyloid-Induced Neurotoxicity and Tau Phosphorylation," *Journal of Ethnopharmacology* 133, no. 3 (2011): 1109–16.

74. C. Wei et al., "Ginsenoside Rg1 Attenuates Beta-Amyloid-Induced Apoptosis in Mutant PS1 M146L Cells," *Neuroscience Letters* 443, no. 3 (2008): 145–9.

75. Y. H. Xie, ["Ginsenoside Rb1 Attenuates Beta-Amyloid Peptide(25-35)-Induced Hyperphosphorylation of Tau Protein Through CDK5 Signal Pathway,"]. *Yao Xue Xue Bao* 42, no. 8 (2007): 828–32 [in Chinese].

76. Z. N. Ji et al., "Ginsenoside Re Attenuate Beta-Amyloid and Serum-Free Induced Neurotoxicity in PC12 Cells," *Journal of Ethnopharmacology* 107, no. 1 (2006): 48–52.

77. F. Chen, E. A. Eckman, and C. B. Eckman, "Reductions in Levels of the Alzheimer's Amyloid Beta Peptide after Oral Administration of Ginsenosides," *The FASEB Journal* 20, no. 8 (2006): 1269–71.

78. N. Li et al., "Protective Effects of Ginsenoside Rg2 against Glutamate-Induced Neurotoxicity in PC12 Cells," *Journal of Ethnopharmacology* 111, no. 3 (2007): 458–63.

79. S. S. Joo and D. I. Lee, "Potential Effects of Microglial Activation Induced by Ginsenoside Rg3 in Rat Primary Culture: Enhancement of Type A Macrophage Scavenger Receptor Expression," *Archives of Pharmacal Research* 28, no. 10 (2005): 1164–9.

80. H. Zhao et al., "Long-Term Ginsenoside Consumption Prevents Memory Loss in Aged SAMP8 Mice by Decreasing Oxidative Stress and Up-Regulating the Plasticity-Related Proteins in Hippocampus," *Brain Research* 1256 (2009): 111–22.

81. C. Tohda, 2004. "Abeta(25-35)-Induced Memory Impairment, Axonal Atrophy, and Synaptic Loss Are Ameliorated by M1, a Metabolite of Protopanaxadiol-Type Saponins," *Neuropsychopharmacology* 29, no. 5 (2004): 860–8.

82. L. Parnetti, F. Amenta, and V. Gallai, "Choline Alphoscerate in Cognitive Decline and in Acute Cerebrovascular Disease: An Analysis of Published Clinical Data," *Mechanics of Ageing and Development* 122, no. 16 (2001): 2041–55.

83. M. De Jesus Moreno Moreno, "Cognitive Improvement in Mild to Moderate Alzheimer's Dementia after Treatment with the Acetylcholine Precursor Choline Alphoscerate:

A Multicenter, Double-Blind, Randomized, Placebo-Controlled Trial," *Clinical Therapeutics* 25, no. 1 (2003): 178–93.

84. Y. T. Choi et al., 2001. "The Green Tea Polyphenol (-) Epigallocatechin Gallate Attenuates Beta-Amyloid-Induced Neurotoxicity in Cultured Hippocampal Neurons," *Life Sciences* 70 (2001): 603–14.

85. S. J. Kim et al., "Epigallocatechin-3-Gallate Suppresses NF-kappaB Activation and Phosphorylation of p38 MAPK and JNK in Human Astrocytoma U373MG Cells," *The Journal of Nutritional Biochemistry* 18 (2007): 587–96.

86. M. Singh et al., "Challenges for Research on Polyphenols from Foods in Alzheimer's Disease: Bioavailability, Metabolism, and Cellular and Molecular Mechanisms," *Journal of Agricultural and Food Chemistry* 56 (2008): 4855–73.

87. K. Rezai-Zadeh et al., 2005. "Green Tea Epigallocatechin-3-gallate (EGCG) Modulates Amyloid Precursor Protein Cleavage and Reduces Cerebral Amyloidosis in Alzheimer Transgenic Mice," *The Journal of Neuroscience* 25: 8807–14.

88. S. Y. Jeon et al., "Green Tea Catechins as a BACE1 (Beta-Secretase) Inhibitor," *Bioorganic & Medicinal Chemistry Letters* 13 (2003): 3905–8.

89. K. Ono et al., "Potent Anti-Amyloidogenic and Fibril-Destabilizing Effects of Polyphenols In Vitro: Implications for the Prevention and Therapeutics of Alzheimer's Disease," *Journal of Neurochemistry* 87 (2003): 172–81.

90. A. M. Haque et al., "Green Deficits Tea Catechins Prevent Cognitive Caused by Abeta1-40 in Rats," *The Journal of Nutritional Biochemistry* 19 (2008): 619–26.

91. S. Y. Lee et al., "Effects of Delayed Administration of (-)-Epigallocatechin Gallate, A Green Tea Polyphenol on the Changes in Polyamine Levels and Neuronal Damage after Transient Forebrain Ischemia in Gerbils," *Brain Research Bulletin* 61 (2003): 399–406.

92. S. T. Henderson, "Ketone Bodies as a Therapeutic for Alzheimer's Disease," *Neurotherapeutics* 5, no. 3 (2008): 470–80.

93. M. A. Reger et al., "Effects of Beta-Hydroxybutyrate on Cognition in Memory-Impaired Adults," *Neurobiology of Aging* 25, no. 3 (2004): 311–4.

94. R. D. Feinman, "Intention-to-Treat: What is the Question?" *Nutrition & Metabolism* 6 (2009): 1.

95. I. Van der Auwera et al., "A Ketogenic Diet Reduces Amyloid Beta 40 and 42 in a Mouse Model of Alzheimer's Disease," *Nutrition & Metabolism* 2 (2005): 28.

96. M. Gasior, M. A. Rogawski, and A. L. Hartman. "Neuroprotective and Disease-Modifying Effects of the Ketogenic Diet," *Behavioural Pharmacology* 17, no. 5–6 (2006): 431–9.

97. P. Lu et al., 2009. "Silibinin Attenuates Amyloid Beta(25-35) Peptide-Induced Memory Impairments: Implication of Inducible Nitric-Oxide Synthase and Tumor Necrosis Factor-Alpha In Mice," *The Journal of Pharmacology and Experimental Therapeutics* 331, no. 1 (2009): 319–26.

98. P. Lu et al., "Silibinin Prevents Amyloid Beta Peptide-Induced Memory Impairment and Oxidative Stress in Mice," *British Journal of Pharmacology* 157, no. 7 (2009): 1270–7.

99. N. Murata et al., "Silymarin Attenuated the Amyloid β Plaque Burden and Improved Behavioral Abnormalities in an Alzheimer's Disease Mouse Model," *Bioscience, Biotechnology, and Biochemistry* 74, no. 11 (2010): 2299–306.

100. P. I. Moreira et al., "Lipoic Acid and N-Acetyl Cysteine Decrease Mitochondrial-Related Oxidative Stress in Alzheimer Disease Patient Fibroblasts," *Journal of Alzheimer's Disease* 12, no. 2 (2007): 195–206.

101. J. C. Adair, J. E. Knoefel, and N. Morgan, "Controlled Trial of N-Acetylcysteine for Patients with Probable Alzheimer's Disease," *Neurology* 57, no. 8 (2001): 1515–7.

102. A. Chan et al., "Efficacy of a Vitamin/Nutriceutical Formulation of Early-Stage Alzheimer's Disease: A 1-Year, Open-Label Pilot Study with a 16-Month Caregiver Extension," *American Journal of Alzheimer's Disease and Other Dementias* 23, no. 6 (2008): 571–85.

103. A. McCaddon and P. R. Hudson, "L-Methylfolate, Methylcobalamin, and N-Acetylcysteine in the Treatment of Alzheimer's Disease-Related Cognitive Decline," *CNS Spectrums* 15, 1 Suppl. 1 (2010): 2–5. Discussion. 6.

104. N. D. Riediger et al., "A Systemic Review of the Roles of N-3 Fatty Acids in Health and Disease," *Journal of the American Dietetic Association* 109, no. 4 (2009): 668–79.

105. R. P. Friedland, "Fish Consumption and the Risk of Alzheimer Disease: Is It Time to Make Dietary Recommendations?" *Archives of Neurology* 60, no. 7 (2003): 923–4.

106. G. A. Jicha and W. R. Markesbery. "Omega-3 Fatty Acids: Potential Role in the Management of Early Alzheimer's Disease," *Clinical Interventions in Aging* 5 (2010): 45–61.

107. G. M. Cole and S. A. Frautschy, "DHA May Prevent Age-Related Dementia," *The Journal of Nutrition* 140, no. 4 (2010): 869–74.

108. T. Crook et al., "Effects of Phosphatidylserine in Alzheimer's Disease," *Psychopharmacology Bulletin* 28, no. 1 (1992): 61–6.

109. T. H. Crook et al., "Effects of Phosphatidylserine in Age-Associated Memory Impairment," *Neurology* 41, no. 5 (1991): 644–9.

110. P. J. Delwaide et al., 1986. "Double-Blind Randomized Controlled Study of Phosphatidylserine in Senile Demented Patients," *Acta Neurologica Scandinavica* 73, no. 2 (1986): 136–40.

111. W. D. Heiss et al., 1994. "Long-Term Effects Of Phosphatidylserine, Pyritinol, and Cognitive Training in Alzheimer's Disease: A Neuropsychological, EEG, and PET Investigation," *Dementia* 5, no. 2 (1994): 88–98.

112. T. Cenacchi et al., "Cognitive Decline in the Elderly: A Double-Blind, Placebo-Controlled Multicenter Study on Efficacy of Phosphatidylserine Administration," *Aging (Milano)* 5, no. 2 (1993): 123–33.

113. R. R. Engel et al., "Double-Blind Cross-Over Study of Phosphatidylserine vs. Placebo in Patients with Early Dementia of the Alzheimer Type," *European Neuropsychopharmacology* 2, no. 2 (1992): 149–55.

114. S. Schreiber et al., "An Open Trial of Plant-Source Derived Phosphatydilserine [sic] for Treatment of Age-Related Cognitive Decline," *The Israel Journal of Psychiatry and Related Sciences* 37 (2000): 302–7.

115. H. Y. Kim et al., "Inhibition of Neuronal Apoptosis by Docosahexaenoic Acid (22:6n-3): Role of Phosphatidylserine in Antiapoptotic Effect," *The Journal of Biological Chemistry* 275 (2000): 35215–23.

116. M. Harwood et al., "A Critical Review of the Data Related to the Safety of Quercetin and Lack of Evidence of In Vivo Toxicity, Including Lack of Genotoxic/Carcinogenic Properties," *Food and Chemical Toxicology* 45 (2007): 2179–205.

117. "Quercetin" *Alternative Medicine Review* 3 (1998): 140–3.

118. A. H. Goldfarb, "What is a True Placebo?" *Medicine and Science in Sports and Exercise* 40, no. 4 (2008): 775. Author reply. 776.

119. S. M. Kuo, P. S. Leavitt, and C. P. Lin. "Dietary Flavonoids Interact with Trace Metals and Affect Metallothionein Level in Human Intestinal Cells," *Biological Trace Element Research* 62 (1998): 135–53.

120. F. Tchantchou et al., "Stimulation of Neurogenesis and Synaptogenesis by Bilobalide and Quercetin via Common Final Pathway in Hippocampal Neurons," *Journal of Alzheimer's Disease* 18, no. 4 (2009): 787–98.

121. M. A. Ansari et al., "Protective Effect of Quercetin in Primary Neurons against Abeta(1-42): Relevance to Alzheimer's Disease," *The Journal of Nutritional Biochemistry* 20, no. 4 (2009): 269–75.

122. A. Tedeschi et al., "Effect of Flavonoids on the Abeta(25-35)-Phospholipid Bilayers Interaction," *European Journal of Medicinal Chemistry* 45, no. 9 (2010): 3998–4003.

123. J. A. Baur et al., "Resveratrol Improves Health and Survival of Mice on a High-Calorie Diet," *Nature* 444, no. 7117 (2006): 337–42.

124. M. Lagouge et al., "Resveratrol Improves Mitochondrial Function and Protects against Metabolic Disease by Activating SIRT1 and PGC-1alpha," *Cell* 127, no. 6 (2006): 1109–22.

125. J. L. Barger et al., "A Low Dose of Dietary Resveratrol Partially Mimics Caloric Restriction and Retards Aging Parameters in Mice," *PLoS One* 3, no. 6 (2008): e2264.

126. C. E. Harper et al., "Resveratrol Suppresses Prostate Cancer Progression in Transgenic Mice," *Carcinogenesis* 28, no. 9 (2007): 1946–53.

127. S. S. Karuppagounder, "Dietary Supplementation with Resveratrol Reduces Plaque Pathology in a Transgenic Model of Alzheimer's Disease," *Neurochemistry International* 54, no. 2 (2009): 111–8.

128. P. Marambaud, H. Zhao, and P. Davies, "Resveratrol Promotes Clearance of Alzheimer's Disease Amyloid-Beta Peptides," *The Journal of Biological Chemistry* 280 (2005): 37377–82.

129. E. Candelario-Jalil et al., 2007. "Resveratrol Potently Reduces Prostaglandin E2 Production and Free Radical Formation in Lipopolysaccharide-Activated Primary Rat Microglia," *Journal of Neuroinflammation* 4: 25.

130. Z. Cao and Y. Li. "Potent Induction of Cellular Antioxidants and Phase 2 Enzymes by Resveratrol in Cardiomyocytes: Protection against Oxidative and Electrophilic Injury," *European Journal of Pharmacology* 489, no. 1–2 (2004): 39–48.

131. A. Kumar et al., "Neuroprotective Effects of Resveratrol against Intracerebroventricular Colchicine-Induced Cognitive Impairment and Oxidative Stress in Rats," *Pharmacology* 79, no. 1 (2007): 17–26.

132. C. A. Oomen et al., "Resveratrol Preserves Cerebrovascular Density and Cognitive Function in Aging Mice," *Frontiers in Aging Neuroscience* 1 (2009): 4.

133. C. R. Gale, C. N. Martyn, and C. Cooper. "Cognitive Impairment and Mortality in a Cohort of Elderly People," *BMJ* 312, no. 7031 (1996): 608–11.

134. W. Wang et al., "Nutritional Biomarkers in Alzheimer's Disease: The Association between Carotenoids, N-3 Fatty

Acids, and Dementia Severity," *Journal of Alzheimer's Disease* 13, no. 1 (2008): 31–8.

135. H. J. Stuerenburg, S. Ganzer, and T. Müller-Thomsen, "Plasma Beta Carotene in Alzheimer's Disease: Association with Cerebrospinal Fluid Beta-Amyloid 1-40, (Abeta40), Beta-Amyloid 1-42 (Abeta42) and Total Tau," *Neuro Endocrinology Letters* 26, no. 6 (2005): 696–8.

136. Z. Zaman et al., "Plasma Concentration of Vitamins A and E and Carotenoids in Alzheimer's Disease," *Age and Ageing* 21, no. 2 (1992): 91–4.

137. E. E. Devore et al., "Dietary Antioxidants and Long-Term Risk of Dementia," *Archives of Neurology* 67, no. 7 (2010): 819–25.

138. M. Fotuhi et al., "Better Cognitive Performance in Elderly Taking Antioxidant Vitamins E and C Supplements in Combination with Nonsteroidal Anti-Inflammatory Drugs: The Cache County Study," *Alzheimer's & Dementia* 4, no. 3 (2008): 223–7.

139. P. P. Zandi, "Reduced Risk of Alzheimer Disease in Users of Antioxidant Vitamin Supplements: The Cache County Study," *Archives of Neurology* 61, no. 1 (2004): 82–8.

140. G. G. Fillenbaum et al., "Dementia and Alzheimer's Disease in Community-Dwelling Elders Taking Vitamin C and/or Vitamin E," *The Annals of Pharmacotherapy* 39, no. 12 (2005): 2009–14.

141. M. B. Isaac, R. Quin, and N. Tabet, 2008. "Vitamin E for Alzheimer's Disease and Mild Cognitive Impairment," *Cochrane Database of Systematic Reviews* 3: CD002854.

142. D. Laurin et al., "Midlife Dietary Intake of Antioxidants and Risk of Late-Life Incident Dementia: The Honolulu-Asia Aging Study," *American Journal of Epidemiology* 159, no. 10 (2004): 959–67.

143. F. J. Jiménez-Jiménez et al., "Serum Levels of Beta-Carotene, Alpha-Carotene and Vitamin A in Patients with Alzheimer's Disease," *European Journal of Neurology* 6, no. 4 (1999): 495–7.

144. M. M. Grant, V. S. Barber, and H. R. Griffiths. "The Presence of Ascorbate Induces Expression of Brain Derived Neurotrophic Factor in SH-SY5Y Neuroblastoma Cells after Peroxide Insult, Which is Associated with Increased Survival," *Proteomics* 5, no. 2 (2005): 534–40.

145. F. E. Harrison et al., "Vitamin C Reduces Spatial Learning Deficits in Middle-Aged and Very Old APP/PSEN1 Transgenic and Wild-Type Mice," *Pharmacology, Biochemistry, and Behavior* 93, no. 4 (2009): 443–50.

146. M. Sano et al., "A Controlled Trial of Selegiline, Alpha-Tocopherol, or Both as Treatment for Alzheimer's Disease: The Alzheimer's Disease Cooperative Study," *The New England Journal of Medicine* 336, no. 17 (1997): 1216–22.

147. S. Sung et al., "Early Vitamin E Supplementation in Young but Not Aged Mice Reduces Abeta Levels and Amyloid Deposition in a Transgenic Model of Alzheimer's Disease," *The FASEB Journal* 18 (2004): 323–5.

148. C. Rota et al., "Dietary Vitamin E Modulates Differential Gene Expression in the Rat Hippocampus: Potential Implications for its Neuroprotective Properties," *Nutritional Neuroscience* 8 (2005): 21–9.

149. L. A. Boothby and P. L. Doering, "Vitamin C and Vitamin E for Alzheimer's Disease," *The Annals of Pharmacotherapy* 39, no. 12 (2005): 2073–80.

150. B. Wolozin, "Simvastatin is Associated with a Reduced Incidence of Dementia and Parkinson's Disease," *BMC Medicine* 5 (2007): 20.

151. R. G. Riekse et al., "Effect of Statins on Alzheimer's Disease Biomarkers in Cerebrospinal Fluid," *Journal of Alzheimer's Disease* 10, no. 4 (2006): 399–406.

152. K. M. Sink et al., "Angiotensin-Converting Enzyme Inhibitors and Cognitive Decline in Older Adults with Hypertension: Results from the Cardiovascular Health Study," *Archives of Internal Medicine* 169, no. 13 (2009): 1195–202.

153. T. Ohrui et al., "Effects of Brain-Penetrating ACE Inhibitors on Alzheimer Disease Progress," *Neurology* 63, no. 7 (2004): 1324–5.

154. I. M. Hajjar et al., "Angiotensin Converting Enzyme Inhibitors and Cognitive and Functional Decline in Patients with Alzheimer's Disease: An Observational Study," *American Journal of Alzheimer's Disease and Other Dementias* 23, no. 1 (2008): 77–83.

155. N. Hirawa et al., "Longer-Term Inhibition of Renin-Angiotensin System Sustains Memory Function in Aged Dahl Rats," *Hypertension* 34, no. 3 (1999): 496–502.

156. N. C. Li et al., "Use of Angiotensin Receptor Blockers and Risk of Dementia in a Predominantly Male Population: Prospective Cohort Analysis," *BMJ* 340 (2010): b5465.

References for Step 5: Maintaining Healthy Hormone Levels

1. K. Yaffe et al., "Sex Hormones and Cognitive Function in Older Men," *Journal of the American Geriatrics Society* 50, no. 4 (2002): 707–12.

2. E. Barrett-Connor, D. Goodman-Gruen, and B. Patay, "Endogenous Sex Hormones and Cognitive Function in

Older Men," *The Journal of Clinical Endocrinology and Metabolism* 84, no. 10 (1999): 3681–5.

3. M. M. Cherrier et al., "Characterization of Verbal and Spatial Memory Changes from Moderate to Supraphysiological Increases in Serum Testosterone in Healthy Older Men," *Psychoneuroendocrinology* 32, no. 1 (2007): 72–9.

4. M. M. Cherrier et al., "Testosterone Improves Spatial Memory in Men with Alzheimer Disease and Mild Cognitive Impairment," *Neurology* 64, no. 12 (2005): 2063–8.

5. G. Verdile et al., "Luteinizing Hormone Levels Are Positively Correlated with Plasma Amyloid-Beta Protein Levels in Elderly Men," *Journal of Alzheimer's Disease* 14, no. 2 (2008): 201–8.

6. M. Yao et al., "Androgens Regulate Neprilysin Expression: Role in Reducing Beta-Amyloid Levels," *Journal of Neurochemistry* 105, no. 6 (2008): 2477–88.

7. H. Q. Yang et al., ["Effect of Estrogen-Depletion And 17beta-Estradiol Replacement Therapy upon Rat Hippocampus Beta-Amyloid Generation,"] *Zhonghua Yi Xue Za Zhi* 89, no. 37 (2009): 2658–61 [in Chinese].

8. G. K. Gouras et al., "Testosterone Reduces Neuronal Secretion of Alzheimer's Beta-Amyloid Peptides," *Proceedings of the National Academy of Sciences of the United States of America* 97, no. 3 (2000): 1202–5.

9. S. Y. Park et al., "Caspase-3- and Calpain-Mediated Tau Cleavage Are Differentially Prevented by Estrogen and Testosterone in Beta-Amyloid-Treated Hippocampal Neurons," *Neuroscience* 144, no. 1 (2007): 119–27.

10. Y. Zhang et al., "Estrogen and Androgen Protection of Human Neurons against Intracellular Amyloid Beta1-42

Toxicity through Heat Shock Protein 70," *The Journal of Neuroscience* 24, no. 23 (2004): 5315–21.

11. S. Zhang et al., "Estrogen Stimulates Release of Secreted Amyloid Precursor Protein from Primary Rat Cortical Neurons via Protein Kinase C Pathway," *Acta Pharmacologica Sinica* 26, no. 2 (2005): 171–6.

12. L. Zhao et al., "17β-Estradiol Regulates Insulin-Degrading Enzyme Expression via and ERβ/PI3-K Pathway in Hippocampus: Relevance to Alzheimer's Prevention," *Neurobiology of Aging* 32, no. 11 (2011): 1949–63.

13. Y. P. Tang et al., "Estrogen Increases Brain Expression of the mRNA Encoding Transthyretin, an Amyloid Beta Scavenger Protein," *Journal of Alzheimer's Disease* 6, no. 4 (2004): 413–20. Discussion. 443–9.

14. P. Schönknecht et al., "Reduced Cerebrospinal Fluid Estradiol Levels Are Associated with Increased Beta-Amyloid Levels in Female Patients with Alzheimer's Disease," *Neuroscience Letters* 307, no. 2 (2001): 122–4.

15. K. Yaffe et al., "Endogenous Sex Hormone Levels and Risk of Cognitive Decline in an Older Biracial Cohort," *Neurobiology of Aging* 28, no. 2 (2007): 171–8.

16. A. Valen-Sendstad et al., "Effects of Hormone Therapy on Depressive Symptoms and Cognitive Functions in Women with Alzheimer Disease: A 12 Month Randomized, Double-Blind, Placebo-Controlled Study of Low-Dose Estradiol and Norethisterone," *American Journal of Geriatric Psychiatry* 18, no. 1 (2010): 11–20.

17. M. M. Cherrier, "The Role of Aromatization in Testosterone Supplementation: Effects on Cognition in Older Men," *Neurology* 64, no. 2 (2005): 290–6.

18. J. C. Carroll et al., "Continuous and Cyclic Progesterone Differentially Interact with Estradiol in the Regulation of Alzheimer-like Pathology in Female 3xTransgenic-Alzheimer's Disease Mice," *Endocrinology* 151, no. 6 (2010): 2713–22.

19. C. A. Frye and A. A. Walf, "Progesterone Reduces Depression-Like Behavior in a Murine Model of Alzheimer's Disease" *Age (Dordrecht, Netherlands)* 31, no. 2 (2009): 143–53.

20. P. K. Jodhka et al., "The Differences in Neuroprotective Efficacy of Progesterone and Medroxyprogesterone Acetate Correlate with their Effects on Brain-Derived Neurotrophic Factor Expression," *Endocrinology* 150, no. 7 (2009): 3162–8.

21. J. C. Carroll et al., "Progesterone and Estrogen Regulate Alzheimer-Like Neuropathology in Female 3xTg-AD Mice," *The Journal of Neuroscience* 27, no. 48 (2007): 13357–65.

22. J. B. Hoppe et al., 2010. "Amyloid-Beta Neurotoxicity in Organotypic Culture is Attenuated by Melatonin: Involvement of GSK-3beta, Tau and Neuroinflammation," *Journal of Pineal Research* 48 (3): 230–8.

23. T. García et al., "Protective role of Melatonin on Oxidative Stress Status and RNA Expression in Cerebral Cortex and Cerebellum of AbetaPP Transgenic Mice after Chronic Exposure to Aluminum," *Biological Trace Element Research* 135, no. 1–3 (2010): 220–32.

24. M. J. Jou et al., "Visualization of the Antioxidative Effects of Melatonin at the Mitochondrial Level during Oxidative Stress-Induced Apoptosis of Rat Brain Astrocytes," *Journal of Pineal Research* 37, no. 1 (2004): 55–70.

25. X. Wang, "The Antiapoptotic Activity of Melatonin in Neurodegenerative Diseases," *CNS Neuroscience & Therapeutics* 15, no. 4 (2009): 345–57.

26. M. Tajes et al., "Anti-Aging Properties of Melatonin in an In Vitro Murine Senescence Model: Involvement of the Sirtuin 1 Pathway," *Journal of Pineal Research* 47, no. 3 (2009): 228–37.

27. W. Dong et al., "Differential Effects of Melatonin on Amyloid-Beta Peptide 25-35-Induced Mitochondrial Dysfunction in Hippocampal Neurons at Different States of Culture," *Journal of Pineal Research* 48, no. 2 (2010): 117–25.

28. M. F. Holick et al., "Vitamin D Deficiency," *The New England Journal of Medicine* 357, no. 3 (2007): 266–81.

29. A. Masoumi et al., "1alpha,25-dihydroxyvitamin D3 Interacts with Curcuminoids to Stimulate Amyloid-Beta Clearance by Macrophages of Alzheimer's Disease Patients," *Journal of Alzheimer's Disease* 17, no. 3 (2009): 703–17.

30. C. Annweiler et al., "Dietary Intake of Vitamin D and Cognition in Older Women: A Large Population-Based Study," *Neurology* 75, no. 20 (2010): 1810–6.

31. M. L. Evatt et al., "Prevalence of Vitamin D Insufficiency in Patients with Parkinson Disease and Alzheimer Disease," *Archives of Neurology* 65, no. 10 (2008): 1348–52.

32. F. Magri et al., "Association Between Changes in Adrenal Secretion and Cerebral Morphometric Correlates in Normal Aging and Senile Dementia," *Dementia and Geriatric Cognitive Disorders* 11, no. 2 (2000): 90–9.

33. S. B. Solerte et al., "Dehydroepiandrosterone Sulfate Decreases the Interleukin-2-Mediated Overactivity of the Natural Killer Cell Compartment in Senile Dementia of the Alzheimer Type," *Dementia and Geriatric Cognitive Disorders* 10, no. 1 (1999): 21–7.

34. L. Li et al., "DHEA Prevents Aβ25-35-impaired Survival of Newborn Neurons in the Dentate Gyrus through a Modulation of PI3K-Akt-mTOR Signaling," *Neuropharmacology* 59, 4–5 (2010): 323–33.

35. M. Kato-Negishi and M. Kawahara, "Neurosteroids Block the Increase in Intracellular Calcium Level Induced by Alzheimer's β-Amyloid Protein in Long-Term Cultured Rat Hippocampal Neurons," *Neuropsychiatric Disease and Treatment* 4, no. 1 (2008): 209–18.

36. S. A. Farr et al., "DHEAS Improves Learning and Memory in Aged SAMP8 Mice but Not in Diabetic Mice," *Life Sciences* 75, no. 23 (2004): 2775–85.

37. S. B. Solerte et al., "Decreased Release of the Angiogenic Peptide Vascular Endothelial Growth Factor in Alzheimer's Disease: Recovering Effect with Insulin and DHEA Sulfate," *Dementia and Geriatric Cognitive Disorders* 19, no. 1 (2005): 1–10.

38. M. Schumacher et al., "Steroid Hormones and Neurosteroids in Normal and Pathological Aging of the Nervous System," *Progress in Neurobiology* 71, no. 1 (2003): 3–29.

39. E. Tamagno et al., "Dehydroepiandrosterone Reduces Expression and Activity of BACE in NT2 Neurons Exposed to Oxidative Stress," *Neurobiology of Disease* 14, no. 2 (2003): 291–301.

40. S. Yamada et al., "Effects of Dehydroepiandrosterone Supplementation on Cognitive Function and Activities of Daily Living in Older Women with Mild to Moderate Cognitive Impairment," *Geriatrics & Gerontology International* 10, no. 4 (2010): 280–7.

41. T. D. Parsons et al., "Dhea Supplementation and Cognition in Postmenopausal Women," *The International Journal of Neuroscience* 116, no. 2 (2006): 141–55.

42. D. Kritz-Silverstein et al., "Effects of Dehydroepiandrosterone Supplementation on Cognitive Function and Quality of Life: The DHEA and Well-Ness (DAWN) Trial," *Journal of the American Geriatrics Society* 56, no. 7 (2008): 1292–8.

References for Step 6: Improve Your Brain Power

1. Y. Stern, "Cognitive Reserve and Alzheimer Disease," *Alzheimer's Disease and Associated Disorders* 20, no. 3 Suppl. 2 (2006): S69–74.

2. M. C. Carlson et al., "Midlife Activity Predicts Risk of Dementia in Older Male Twin Pairs," *Alzheimer's & Dementia* 4, no. 5 (2008): 324–31.

3. L. Fratiglioni and H. X. Wang. "Brain Reserve Hypothesis in Dementia," *Journal of Alzheimer's Disease* 12, no. 1 (2007): 11–22.

4. A. Acevedo and D. A. Loewenstein, "Nonpharmacological Cognitive Interventions in Aging and Dementia," *Journal of Geriatric Psychiatry and Neurology* 20, no. 4 (2007): 239–49.

5. J. P. Zhou et al., "Transduced PTD-BDNF Fusion Protein Protects against Beta Amyloid Peptide-Induced Learning and Memory Deficits in Mice," *Brain Research* 1191 (2008): 12–9.

6. S. Arancibia et al., "Protective Effect of BDNF against Beta-Amyloid Induced Neurotoxicity In Vitro and In Vivo in Rats," *Neurobiology of Disease* 31, no. 3 (2008): 316–26.

7. A. Moore and P. Malinowski, "Meditation, Mindfulness and Cognitive Flexibility," *Consciousness and Cognition* 18, no. 1 (2009): 176–86.

8. F. Zeidan et al., "Mindfulness Meditation Improves Cognition: Evidence of Brief Mental Training," *Consciousness and Cognition* 19, no. 2 (2010): 597–605.

9. A. Chiesa, R. Calati, and A. Serretti. "Does Mindfulness Training Improve Cognitive Abilities? A Systematic Review of Neuropsychological Findings," *Clinical Psychology Review* 31, no. 3 (2011): 449–64.

10. P. A. van den Hurk et al., "Greater Efficiency in Attentional Processing Related to Mindfulness Meditation," *Quarterly Journal of Experimental Psychology* 63, no. 6 (2010): 1168–80.

11. S. W. Lazar and B. Fischl. "Meditation Experience is Associated with Increased Cortical Thickness," *Neuroreport* 16, no. 17 (2005): 1893–7.

12. A. Karp et al., "Mental, Physical and Social Components in Leisure Activities Equally Contribute to Decrease Dementia Risk," *Dementia and Geriatric Cognitive Disorders* 21, no. 2 (2006): 65–73.

13. G. Rauchs et al., "Is There a Link between Sleep Changes and Memory in Alzheimer's Disease?" *Neuroreport* 19, no. 11 (2008): 1159–62.

14. G. Rauchs et al., ["Sleep and Episodic Memory: A Review of the Literature in Young Healthy Subjects and Potential Links between Sleep Changes and Memory Impairment Observed during Aging and Alzheimer's Disease,"] *Revue neurologique* (*Paris*) 166, no. 11 (2010): 873–81. [in French].

15. S. Kim et al., "Neurocognitive Dysfunction Associated with Sleep Quality and Sleep Apnea in Patients with Mild Cognitive Impairment," *American Journal of Geriatrics and Psychiatry* 19, no. 4 (2011): 374–81.

16. Y. Huang et al., "Effects of Age and Amyloid Deposition on aβ Dynamics in the Human Central Nervous System," *Archives of Neurology* 69, no. 1 (2012): 51–8.

17. J. E. Kang et al., "Amyloid-Beta Dynamics are Regulated by Orexin and the Sleep-Wake Cycle," *Science* 326, no. 5955 (2009): 1005–7.

18. D. A. Weldemichael and G. T. Grossberg. 2010. "Circadian Rhythm Disturbances in Patients with Alzheimer's Disease: A Review," *International Journal of Alzheimer's Disease* pii: 716453.

19. David Rakel, "Improving and Maintaining a Healthy Sleep-Wake Cycle." University of Wisconsin-Madison, Department of Family Medicine. Accessed January 22, 2012. http://www.fammed.wisc.edu/sites/default/files//webfm-uploads/documents/outreach/im/handout_sleep.pdf.

References for the Appendix

1. P. Y Scarabin et al., "Differential Association of Oral and Transdermal Oestrogen-Replacement Therapy with Venous Thromboembolism Risk," *The Lancet* 362, no. 9382 (2003): 428–32.

2. K. Holtorf, "The Bioidentical Hormone Debate: Are Bioidentical Hormones (Estradiol, Estriol, and Progesterone) Safer or More Efficacious than Commonly Used Synthetic Versions in Hormone Replacement Therapy?" *Postgraduate Medicine* 121, no. 1 (2009): 73–85.

3. M. K. Kim and J. H. Park, "Conference on "Multidisciplinary Approaches to Nutritional Problems." Symposium on "Nutrition and Health." Cruciferous Vegetable Intake and the Risk of Human Cancer: Epidemiological Evidence," *The Proceedings of the Nutrition Society* 68, no. 1 (2009): 103–10.

Index

A

abdominal breathing, 116

Aceon (perindopril), 83

acetylcholine (neurotransmitter), 4, 70–72, 81, 123

acetyl-l-carnitine, 60–61, 76, 86

AD. *See* Alzheimer's disease (AD)

advanced glycation end products (AGEs), 38–39, 80

aerobic training, 45–46

age-related

    Alzheimer's, 73

    degenerative diseases, 40

    diseases, 37, 127

    memory impairment, 71

AGEs. *See* advanced glycation end products (AGEs)

air pollution, 31, 36

alcohol, 113

alpha-lipoic acid (antioxidant), 33–34, 61–62, 86

alpha-secretase, 72

alpha-tocopherol (vitamin E), 33–34, 76, 80–81, 86

ALS. *See* Lou Gehrig's disease (ALS)

alum, 21–22

aluminum, 21–22

Alzheimer's dementia, 3

Alzheimer's disease (AD). *See also* avenues to Alzheimer's disease; beta-amyloid plaque; dementia; neurofibrillary tangles; supplements; tau protein

age-related, 73

alpha-lipoic acid and, 61–62

behavior, irritable, obstinate and combative, 14

beta-amyloid plaque and neurofibrillary tangles work together to kill brain cells in, 16

brain atrophy (shrinking) in, 16, 20, 39, 79

brain biochemistry, multifaceted approach to, 4–5

brain-cell death, 16, 20, 37–39, 64, 69, 71

causes, many, 4

daily living tasks, difficulty with, 14

death, sixth leading cause of, 15

depression and, 14

DHEA benefits, 98
disease progression, slowing, 13
disease progression without
    adequate treatment, 14–15
estradiol benefits, 92–94
executive function, loss of, 14
FDA-approved medications for,
    4–5, 81–82
genetically transmitted form of,
    73–74
hormones and, 89–96
instigators of, influencing two,
    59–60
key processes in, 58–60
melatonin benefits, 96–97
progesterone benefits, 94–95
root causes of, therapy
    addressing, 6, 35
short-term memory, loss of, 14,
    77
single drug cure, there is no, 17
testosterone benefits, 90
vitamin D3 benefits, 98
American ginseng, 70–71
amyloid precursor protein (APP),
    58, 91, 100
amyloid toxicity, 9, 30
amyotrophic lateral sclerosis (ALS),
    74, 97
Amyvid PET scan, 2–3
anti-Alzheimer avenues
    about, 5–7
    avenues as supply routes for
        nurturing and improving
        your brain, 5
antiglycating (blood sugar control),
    52
anti-glycating nutritional
    supplement, 56
anti-inflammatory, 52
antioxidants, 33–36, 52
antioxidant supplements, 34–36
antiperspirants, 21
APO E1, E2, E3 genotypes, 73–74
APOE4 genotype, 73–74

apoptosis. *See* cell death
APP. *See* amyloid precursor protein
    (APP)
arborization (brain-cell branching),
    103
Aristotle, 2
artichokes, 29
aspartame (sweetener), 42
aspirin, 85
attentional capacity, 107
avenues to Alzheimer's disease
    avenue 1: oxidative stress, 7
    avenue 2: glycation, 7–8
    avenue 3: inflammation, 8
    avenue 4: beta-amyloid protein
        production in brain, 8
    avenue 5: beta-amyloid protein
        elimination in brain, 8–9
    avenue 6: beta-amyloid toxicity
        and destruction of brain
        cells, 9, 30
    avenue 7: abnormal tau protein,
        9
    avenue 8: cognitive function
        enhancement, 10
    avenue 9: brain plasticity
        improvement, 10
Axona (prescription), 73

B
baby-boomer population, 15
baked goods, 41–42
baking powder, 21
bananas, 14, 43, 48
BDNF. *See* brain-derived
    neurotrophic factor (BDNF)
beans, 29–30, 42
bedroom, 114
beets, 44, 48
beta-amyloid plaque. *See also*
    neurofibrillary tangles
    Alzheimer's disease and, 2–3,
        39, 58–59, 64
    American ginseng and, 71
    brain autopsy and, 16

brain cells killed by
neurofibrillary tangles and,
16
curcumin and, 68
elevated homocysteine and low
B-vitamin levels and, 64
ginger and, 70
neurofibrillary tangles and,
16–17, 58
resveratrol and, 79
sleep and, 111
testosterone and, 90
vitamin D and, 97
beta-amyloid protein
amyloid precursor protein
(APP), from cleavage of, 91
elimination of, in the brain, 8–9
free radical formation,
increases, 20
metals interact with, 29
oxidation (brain-cell "rusting"),
causes, 16
phosphorylation of tau protein
and, 29–30
production of, in the brain, 8
toxicity and destruction of brain
cells, 9
what it is, and what it does,
15–16
beta-amyloid toxicity, 9, 30
beta carotene (antioxidant), 33–34,
80–81, 86
beta-hydroxybutyrate, 74
beta-secretase, 58, 72, 91, 98, 100
BHRT. *See* Bioidentical Hormone
Replacement Therapy
(BHRT)
bioflavonoids, 78, 86
Bioidentical Hormone Replacement
Therapy (BHRT), 94, 120,
131, 134
BHRT *vs.* WHI therapy, 131134
myths about, 129–31
science of hormone molecules,
131

Women's Health Initiative
(WHI), 130–33
bioidentical hormones, 5
bioidentical progesterone, 95. *See
also* progesterone
blood-brain barrier, 82–83
blood clots, 132
blood donation, 36
blood pressure, elevated, 108
blood pressure medications, 84
blood sugar level, 39–40
bluefish grouper, 23
board games, 104
bone-building hormone, 95. *See also*
progesterone
bone density, 47
Boreham, Dr., 51
boron, 55
brain, normal, 2
brain aerobics, 103–6, 117
brain atrophy (shrinking), 16, 20,
39, 79
brain-cell(s)
function of, 9, 73
growth of, 45
mitochondria, 97
brain cell death. *See also* cell death
(apoptosis); hippocampus;
inflammation
American ginseng fights
formation of beta amyloid
and NFTs, 71
beta amyloid, cleavage of tau
and, 69
beta-amyloid toxicity and, 9
biochemical events leading to
plaques and, 5
elevated protein and lipid
oxidation, 69
ginger and free radicals, 70
meditation and brain's cortex, 108
in memory area of brain, 16
neuroprotection from
ketone bodies and beta-
hydroxybutyrate, 74

oxidative stress and, 7, 20, 64
phosphatidylserine to prevent, 76–77
brain-cell "rusting," 16. *See also* oxidative stress
brain-derived neurotrophic factor (BDNF), 45, 77, 104
brain scan. See Amyvid PET scan
brain vasculature (blood-flow network), 108
bran breads, 42
bran cereal, 42
breast cancer, 132–34
breathing exercises, 113–14
bright-light therapy, 112. *See also* sleep
British Medical Journal, 84
broccoli extract, 55
brown rice, 42

C

cadmium (toxic metal), 29. *See also* phytate
caffeine, 65–67
calcium, 27, 30, 36
calcium (supplement), 27, 55
calcium channels in cell, 99
Camellia senensis (tea plant), 72
cancer, 72, 76, 108
    breast, 132–34
    endometrial, 94–95
    prevention, 55, 72, 134
candesartan (Atacand), 84
candy, 41
captopril (Capoten), 83
carbohydrates, 41, 43
carbo-loading, 39
card games, 104
cardiovascular disease, 46, 78–79
carrots, 44, 48
celecoxib (Celebrex), 85
cell death (apoptosis). *See also* brain cell death
    American ginseng and, 70
    in area used for memory, 16

beta amyloid and cleavage of tau protein, 69
beta-amyloid plaque induced, 64
ginger and, 70
ketone bodies and beta-hydroxybutyrate, 74
oxidative stress and, 7, 20, 64, 69
phosphatidylserine and, 78
cell phone, 33
cereals, iron-enriched, 28
chicken giblets, 29
chickpeas, 29
cholecalciferol. *See* vitamin D3
choline alfoscerate, 71–72
chronic stress, 89, 108–9
circadian rhythm, 96, 111–12
citrus bioflavonoids, 78, 86
coconut oil, 73, 75, 87
coenzyme Q10 (antioxidant), 33–34
coffee/caffeine, 65–67
cognitive
    activity, 103–4, 109
    difficulty, 2
    exercise, 104–6
    reserve, 104
    testing, professional, 3
cognitive function, 9
    drugs to improve, 84
    enhancement of, 10
    mental exercises for, 105–6
cognitive impairment. *See also* mild cognitive impairment
    acetyl-l-carnitine and, 60
    angiotensin receptor blockers (ARBs), 84
    beta-amyloid toxicity and, 9
    brain aerobics and, 103
    caffeine and, 65–66
    green tea and, 72
    high blood sugar and, 40
    medium chain triglycerides (MCTs) and, 73
    melatonin and, 96
    Six-Step Program and, 123–24

vitamin B3 (nicotinamide) and, 65
vitamin D3 and, 97–98
vitamin E, vitamin C and beta-carotene and, 80–81
conjugated equine estrogen, 132
copper, 26–27, 55
cortex (area of brain), 108
cortisol, 89, 108–9
Cozaar (losartan), 84
crossword puzzles, 103
curcumin (antioxidant), 68
cytokines, 38, 99

D
degenerative disease, 40, 50, 80, 108–9
dehydroepiandrosterone (DHEA), 89–90, 98–101
dementia. *See also* Alzheimer's disease
   acetyl-l-carnitine and, 60–61
   alpha-lipoic acid and, 61–62
   Alzheimer's, 3, 14
   angiotensin-converting enzyme inhibitors (ACEIs), 83
   angiotensin receptor blockers (ARBs), 84
   B12 and, 63
   bioidentical hormone replacement and, 131–32
   brain aerobics and, 103
   chronic stress and, 108–9
   cognitive activity and, 103
   glycation and, 37
   glycerylphosphorylcholine, 71
   high blood pressure and, 84
   high blood sugar and, 40
   homocysteine levels, 63–64, 76
   mindfulness and, 109
   nicotinamide and, 65
   nonsteroidal anti-inflammatory drugs (NSAIDs), 85
   from numerous biochemical and physiological events, 57

   omega-3 fatty acids and, 77
   sleep impairment and, 110
   social activity and, 109
   vascular, 63, 100, 132
dental fillings (amalgams), 26
depression, 14
DHEA. *See* dehydroepiandrosterone (DHEA)
DHT. *See* dihydrotestosterone (DHT)
diabetes, 108
   type II, 40, 65
   type III, 40, 73
dihydrotestosterone (DHT), 91, 101
diindolylmethane (DIM), 55, 134
disease risk, 50
distillation of water, 22, 27, 36
doctor, 4
Donepezil (drug), 111–12
drug companies, 6, 17

E
EGCG. *See* epigallocatechin gallate (EGCG)
egg yolks, 28
electromagnetic radiation (EMR), 33, 36, 113
electrons, 20
EMR. *See* electromagnetic radiation (EMR)
endometrial cancer, 94–95
environmental exposure, 51
environmental factors, 60
epigallocatechin gallate (EGCG), 72–73
epigenetics, 49–51, 53
epigenetic switching, 50
Epigenetic Symphony, 35–36, 53–56, 81, 85. *See also* supplements
epilepsy, 74
epinephrine (adrenaline), 108
estradiol (female hormone), 89–90
estrogen (female hormone). *See also* Bioidentical Hormone

Replacement Therapy
(BHRT)
conjugated equine, 132
oral, 133
replacement, 95, 130
transdermal, 133
in transdermal cream, 133
exercise
Alzheimer's and, 44, 60
blood-sugar control and, 44
cognitive, 104–6
daily, 48
oxidative stress and, 35–36, 45
recommended types of, 45–47
sleep and, 112

F
fats, 41
female hormones, 89, 91, 94. *See
also* estradiol; estrogen;
menopause; progesterone
ferritin levels, 28
ferulic acid, 69
fish
mercury, with high levels of, 23
mercury, with low levels of,
24–25
mercury, with moderate levels
of, 24
fitness coach, 46
flexibility/stretching, 45, 47
foods high in
aluminum, 23–24
copper, 26–27
iron, 28–29
foreign language, 103
fosinopril (Monopril), 83
free radicals. *See also* oxidative stress
beta-amyloid protein increases
formation of, 20
ginger and, 70
neutralizing, 33–34
nitrogen (oxidative stress), 75
oxidative stress, causing, 20,
38, 45

"French paradox," 78–79
fruit
antioxidants and, 43
bioflavonoids in, 78
dried, 28
glycemic index of, 43
health benefits of, 78
juice, 44, 48
low glycemic nutrition and, 41
organic, 32–33
pesticides and, 32

G
gamma secretase, 58, 66
gastric reflux disease, 109
gene expression, 51, 53, 79–80
genetic blueprint, 49–50
ginger (anti-inflammatory), 69–70
glucose metabolism, 73
glutamate toxicity, 71
glutathione (antioxidant), 35, 55, 61,
75–76
glycation. *See also* advanced
glycation end products
(AGEs)
age-related diseases and, 37
Alzheimer's disease and, 7–8
brain cell death from excess,
37–39
carbohydrates and, 43
high blood sugar and, 37
glycemic
index, 42–44
load, reducing, 43
nutrition, low, 40–42
glycerylphosphorylcholine, 71–72
Goethe, Johann Wolfgang von, 1
grains, iron-enriched, 28
greens, dark leafy, 28
green tea, 72–73

H
heart attack, 108, 132
heart disease, 76, 83, 121–22, 134
heart rate, 46, 108

heat-shock protein, 45
hippocampus (memory area of
 brain), 16, 66, 71, 84, 96,
 99, 109. *See also* brain cell
 death
HMG CoA reductase, 82
hobby, intellectually challenging,
 103
homocysteine (amino acid), 62–64,
 76
hormone replacement. *See also*
 Bioidentical Hormone
 Replacement Therapy
 (BHRT)
 about, 53, 94, 101, 120
 after menopause, 94
hormones. *See also* melatonin
 Alzheimer's disease and, 89–96
 men, recommended for, 101
 women, recommended for, 101
horsetail extract (silica), 55
HS Protein 70 (brain-protective
 protein), 92
Huntington's disease, 96–97

I
I3C. *See* indole-3-carbinol (I3C)
ibuprofen, 85
IDE. *See* insulin-degrading enzyme
 (IDE)
IL2. *See* interleukin 2 (IL2)
Illuminate!™, 86
immune system, 8, 38, 109
immunizations, 22
indole-3-carbinol (I3C), 134
inflammation. *See also* brain cell
 death
 aging of body and, 89
 Alzheimer's disease and, 8
 brain cell destruction and, 38,
 99
 chronic diseases and, 38
 cytokines mediate, 99
 ferulic acid's anti-inflammatory
 effects, 69

ginger and, 70
glycation and, 38
melatonin and, 96
milk thistle and, 75
nutritional supplements and, 51
omega-3 fatty acids and, 76–77
oxidation and glycation and,
 59–60
quercitin or mixed bioflavonoids
 and, 78
resveratrol and, 79
insulin (hormone), 40, 89
 function, 77
 resistance, 40, 79, 97
 sensitivity, 60–61
insulin-degrading enzyme (IDE), 9,
 93
insulin-like growth factor I, 80
interleukin 2 (IL2), 99
iron, foods high in, 28–29
iron-deficiency anemia, 28
iron levels, 28–29
irritable bowel syndrome, 109

J
juicing, 44

K
Kabat-Zinn, Jon, 109
ketone bodies, 73–75
kidneys, 32
kiwi fruit, 43, 48

L
The Lancet, 133
lead (toxic metal), 29. *See also*
 phytate
Lemon, Dr., 51
lentils, 29–30
Leonardi Institute. *See also* Six-Step
 Program
 blood ferritin level testing, 28
 comprehensive treatment
 program, 121
 contact information, 125

daily coffee *vs.* caffeine supplements or decaf coffee, 67

Daley, Nathan (MD), 128

homocysteine levels reduction, 62

Leonardi, David (MD), 127

motto: normal is not necessarily optimal, 62

NSAIDs, potential adverse effects to, 85

patients taught to apply new information, 121

progesterone for women who have had hysterectomies, 95

scientific research on AD, review of all, 120

website, 125

LH. *See* luteinizing hormone (LH)

lifestyles, inactive, 39. *See also* exercise

lisinopril (Prinivil or Zestril), 83–84

liver, 29, 32

long-term care facility, 13

losartan (Cozaar), 84

Lou Gehrig's disease (ALS), 74, 97

lovastatin (medication), 82

low-glycemic nutrition, 40–41

luteinizing hormone (LH), 91

M

mackerel (fish), 23

macrophages, 9

magnesium, 27, 30, 36, 55

magnesium amino acid chelate (supplement), 27

magnetic resonance imaging (MRI), 38

male hormones, 89–91. *See also* dehydroepiandrosterone; testosterone

mangoes, 43, 48

marlin (fish), 23

math problems, 104

MCI. *See* mild cognitive impairment (MCI)

McMaster University, 51, 53, 55

MCT oil, 75, 86

MCTs. *See* medium chain triglycerides (MCTs)

meditation, 106, 113–14, 117

medium chain triglycerides (MCTs), 73–75

medroxyprogesterone (synthetic compound), 130–31. *See also* bioidentical progesterone

melatonin, 33, 80, 89–90, 96–97, 101, 111

meloxicam (Mobic), 85

memantine (Namenda), 4, 71, 81

memory

formation (in hippocampus), 109

impairment, age-related, 71

loss, 2–3, 77

short-term, 14, 77

spatial, 91

verbal, 91, 93

working, 67, 107

memory impairment, age-related, 2

menopause, 90, 92, 94, 129. *See also* female hormones

hormone replacement after, 94

mental checklist, 14

mental exercises for cognitive function, 105–6

mercury, 23–26

avoidance, 26

level, serum, 26

vapor, 26

metals. *See* pro-oxidant metals

microglia (immune cells in brain), 58, 66, 71

mild cognitive impairment (MCI), 2–3, 91, 110. *See also* cognitive impairment

milk thistle/silymarin, 75, 87

mindfulness, 106–9

mindfulness sleep-induction technique, 114, 116–17

mitochondria
  alpha-lipoic acid and, 61
  antioxidant molecules and, 35
  APOE4 genotype and, 74
  energy factories within cells,
    52, 60
  free radicals and, 35
  melatonin and, 96–97
  oxidative stress and, 7
  phosphatidylserine and, 77
  resveratrol and, 79
  vitamin B3 (nicotinamide) and,
    63, 65
molecular damage, 20
mollusks, 29
MRI. *See* magnetic resonance
    imaging (MRI)
multimineral, 54, 56
multivitamin, 54, 56
municipal water supplies, 21–22
municipal water treatment, 22

N
n-acetyl cysteine (antioxidant),
    33–34, 62, 76, 87
naproxen, 85
National Library of Medicine, 6
Natural Resources Defense Council
    website, 25
neprilysin (enzyme), 9, 91–92
neurodegenerative diseases, 75, 96
neurofibrillary tangles (NFTs). *See
    also* beta-amyloid plaque
  beta-amyloid plaque and, 16–
    17, 58
  from cleavage of tau protein, 92
  phosphorylation of tau protein
    and, 29–30
  testosterone and, 90
  what it is, and what it does, 16
neuroplasticity, 10, 71, 104
neurotoxins, 32
Newport, Mary, 75
NFTs. *See* neurofibrillary tangles
    (NFTs)

nicotine, 113
nonstarch vegetables, 44
nonsteroidal anti-Inflammatory
    drugs (NSAIDs), 85
norepinephrine, 108
Norwegian University of Science
    and Technology, 82
NSAIDs. *See* nonsteroidal anti-
    Inflammatory drugs
    (NSAIDs)
nutrients, 51
nutrition, low-glycemic, 40–41
nutritional supplements, 5, 49
  copper in, 26–27
nuts, 26

O
oat bran, 30
oatmeal, 42
obesity, 40, 79, 121, 134
omega-3 fatty acids, 76–77, 87
oral estrogen, 133
oral ginseng, 70
oral phytate supplement, 30
orange roughy, 23
organic fruits, 32–34
organic produce, 32–34, 36
organic vegetables, 32–34
organ meats (liver), 26–27
oxidative stress. *See also* free
    radicals
  air pollution and, 31, 36
  Alzheimer's disease and, 7
  electromagnetic radiation
    (EMF) and, 33
  exercise and, 35–36, 45
  free radicals and, 20, 38, 45, 75
  iron promotes, 28
  pesticides and, 32
  reducing, 10–11, 35–36
  water pollution and, 32

P
Panax quinquefolius, 70–71
pancake mixes, 21

papaya, 43, 48
parasympathetic system, 108
Parkinson's disease, 65, 74–75, 96
pasta, 42
PCBs, 25
peas, 42, 44, 48
perindopril (Aceon), 83
personal trainer, 47
pesticides, 32
PET scan, See Amyvid PET scan
phosphatidylserine, 77–78, 87
phosphorylation
    caffeine and, 65–66
    melatonin and, 96
    neurofibrillary tangles and,
        29–30, 58
    omega-3 fatty acids and, 76
    progesterone and, 95
    simvastatin and, 83
    of tau protein, 65
    vitamin B3 (nicotinamide) and,
        63, 65
phytate (inositol hexaphosphate),
    30–31. See also pro-oxidant
    metals
phytate cream, 30, 36, 85, 87
pineal gland, 96
plaque. See beta-amyloid plaque
plaques, 5
plasticity, 10, 71, 104
postmenopausal
    mice study, 95
    women, 93, 95, 100, 130, 133
post-traumatic stress disorder
    (PTSD), 109
potassium, 27, 30, 36, 55
potassium gluconate (supplement),
    27
pre-Alzheimer's, 2
prescription medications, 5
Preventive Medicine Program, 53
processed foods, 21
progesterone (female hormone).
    See also bioidentical
    progesterone; estradiol

about, 94
Alzheimer's, role of in, 94–95
breast-cancer risk and, 133
female hormone, 89
gradual decline in women
    throughout adult life, 90
medroxyprogesterone vs., 130–
    31
progressive muscle relaxation,
    113–16
pro-oxidant metals. See also phytate
    aluminum, 21–22
    copper, 26–27
    iron, 28–29
    mercury, 23–26
proteins, 41
proteomics, 49–50, 53
PTSD. See post-traumatic stress
    disorder (PTSD)
Pure Life (bottled water), 22

Q
quercitin, 78, 87
Quist-Paulsen, Dr., 82

R
Rakel, David, 116
ramipril (Altace), 83
red meat, 28
redox-positive metals, 29
red wine, 79
references
    Bioidentical Hormone
        Replacement Therapy, 170
    brain power, improving your,
        168–70
    genes, making them work in
        your favor, 142–43
    hormone levels, maintaining
        healthy, 162–68
    root causes of Alzheimer's
        disease, combating, 143–62
    "rustproofing," 135–41
    "sticky" protein cells,
        preventing, 141–42

REM sleep, 110
renin-angiotensinaldosterone system, 83
resistance training, 45–47
resveratrol, 78–79, 87
reverse osmosis filter, 22, 27, 32, 36
rice bran, 30
riddles, deciphering, 104
Rollo, Dr., 51
rutin, 78, 87

S

saccharin (sweetener), 42
s-adenosyl-methionine, 76
salmon, farmed, 25
sea bass, 23
seafood, 23–26
scan, PET. See Amyvid PET scan
selenium (antioxidant), 33–34, 87
senile plaques, 29
"senior moments," 2
serum ferritin, 28, 36
serum mercury level, 26
shark, 23
shellfish, 26
short-term memory, 14, 77
Simvastatin (medication), 82–83, 87
sirtuins (gene product), 97
Six-Step Program. See also avenues
    to Alzheimer's disease;
    Leonardi Institute
  antioxidant supplements, 34–35
  benefits of, 123–25
  components of, 123
  Epigenetic Symphony, 35–36,
    53–56, 81, 85
  how it works, 3–4, 122–23
  Leonardi Institute contact
    information, 125
  patient feedback, 120–21
  program with thirty elements, 5,
    10–11
  results depend on your efforts,
    119–20

supply avenues, defending attack
    on and fortifying, 9–10
support from family and friends,
    121–22
"weapons" to prevent, probably
    arrest, and reverse AD, 7
why it works, 4–5
sleep. See also melatonin
  about, 60, 96, 110–17
  achieving optimal, 112–15
  apnea, 110
  beta-amyloid plaque and, 111
  deprivation, 89, 96
  disorders, 111
  exercise and, 112
  impairment and dementia, 110
  REM, 110
  slow-wave, 110–11
  specialist, 117
Smart Water (bottled water), 22
smokers, 81, 133
social activity, 109–10
soda pop, 41, 44
soybeans, 29
spatial memory, 91
starches, 41–43, 48
statins, 82–83
stevia (sugar substitute), 42
"sticky" proteins, 37–38. See also
    advanced glycation end
    products (AGEs)
strength training, 45–47
stress, 60, 108
stretching/flexibility, 45, 47
stroke, 73–74, 76, 108, 132
sucralose (Splenda), 41–42
sugar, 38
supplements. See also Epigenetic
    Symphony
  acetyl-l-carnitine, 60–61, 76, 86
  alpha-lipoic acid, 61–62, 86
  American ginseng, 70–71, 87
  beta carotene (antioxidant),
    33–34, 80–81, 86
  caffeine, 65–67, 87

citrus bioflavonoids, 78, 86
curcumin (antioxidant), 68, 87
ferulic acid, 69, 87
ginger, 69–70, 86
glycerylphosphorylcholine,
    71–72, 87
green tea, 72–73, 87
medium chain triglycerides
    (MCTs), 73–75, 87
milk thistle/silymarin, 75, 87
n-acetyl cysteine, 76, 87
omega-3 fatty acids, 76–77, 87
phosphatidyl serine, 77–78, 87
quercitin, 78, 87
resveratrol, 78–79, 87
rutin, 78, 87
vitamin B3, 55, 62–65, 87
vitamin B6, 62–65, 86
vitamin B12, 62–65, 86
vitamin C (antioxidant), 33–34,
    80, 86
vitamin E (antioxidant), 33–34,
    76, 80–81, 86
sweets, 41, 48
swordfish, 23

T
tangles, 5
tau protein
    Alzheimer's and abnormal, 9
    Alzheimer's and chemically
        altered, 16
    DHEA and, 100
    melatonin and, 96
    metals and phosphorylation of,
        29–30
    progesterone and, 95
    testosterone and, 90
telmisartan (Micardis), 84
temporal lobe, 16
testosterone (male hormone)
    about, 89–93
    replacement, 91–93
    skin cream, topical, 93
tomato juice, 44

tomato products, 26
toxic metals, 29. *See also* pro-
    oxidant metals
trandolapril (Mavik), 83
transdermal estrogen, 133
trans-resveratrol, 79
transthyretin, 9, 93
traumatic brain injury, 74
tuna, 23–24
turkey giblets, 29
type II diabetes, 40, 65
type III diabetes, 40, 73

V
vascular endothelial growth factor
    (VEGF), 99–100
vegetable juices, 44
vegetables
    organic, 32–33
    pesticides and, 32
vegetables, nonstarch, 44
VEGF. *See* vascular endothelial
    growth factor (VEGF)
verbal memory, 91, 93
visuo-spatial processing, 107
vitamin
    B1 (thiamine), 55
    B2 (riboflavin), 55
    B3 (niacin), 55, 62–65, 87
    B6, 62–65, 86
    B12, 62–65, 86
    C (antioxidant), 33–34, 80, 86
    D3 (cholecalciferol), 55, 68, 86,
        89, 97–98, 101
    E (antioxidant), 33–34, 76,
        80–81, 86
    K, 55

W
waffle mixes, 21
water
    distillation of, 22, 27, 36
    municipal water supplies, 21–22
    pipes, copper, 27
    pollution, 32

from reverse osmosis, 22, 27,
    32, 36
watermelon, 43, 48
websites
    ww.glycemicindex.com, 42
    www.airnow.gov, 31
    www.Cycle-Breakers.com, 53,
        86, 125
    www.LeonardiInstitute.com, 125
    www.mendosa.com, 42
    www.nrdc.org/health/effects/
        mercury/guide.asp, 25
weight lifting, 46–47
weight loss, 72
Wherever You Go, There You Are
    (Kabat-Zinn), 109

WHI. *See* Women's Health Initiative
    (WHI)
white blood cells, 8, 38, 69
whole grains, 26
wireless technologies, 33
Women's Health Initiative (WHI),
    130–33
word searching, 2
working memory, 67, 107

X
xylitol (sugar alcohol), 42

Y
yoga, 47, 113–14

Made in the USA
Charleston, SC
27 November 2012

15919353R00102